AMERICAN
ASSOCIATION
of CRITICAL-CARE
NURSES

AACN
Protocols for Practice

Creating
Healing
Environments

Second Edition

Edited by
Nancy C. Molter, RN, MN, PhD
Choctaw Management Services Enterprises
Clinical Research Coordinator Program Manager
US Army Institute of Surgical Research
Fort Sam Houston, Texas

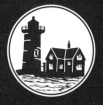

JONES AND BARTLETT PUBLISHERS
Sudbury, Massachusetts
BOSTON   TORONTO   LONDON   SINGAPORE

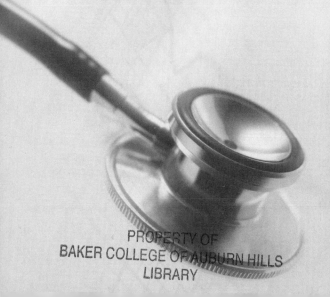

World Headquarters

Jones and Bartlett Publishers
40 Tall Pine Drive
Sudbury, MA 01776
978-443-5000
info@jbpub.com
www.jbpub.com

Jones and Bartlett Publishers Canada
6339 Ormindale Way
Mississauga, Ontario L5V 1J2
CANADA

Jones and Bartlett Publishers International
Barb House, Barb Mews
London W6 7PA
UK

Jones and Bartlett's books and products are available through most bookstores and online booksellers. To contact Jones and Bartlett Publishers directly, call 800-832-0034, fax 978-443-8000, or visit our website, www.jbpub.com.

Substantial discounts on bulk quantities of Jones and Bartlett's publications are available to corporations, professional associations, and other qualified organizations. For details and specific discount information, contact the special sales department at Jones and Bartlett via the above contact information or send an email to specialsales@jbpub.com.

The authors, editor, and publisher have made every effort to provide accurate information. However, they are not responsible for errors, omissions, or for any outcomes related to the use of the contents of this book and take no responsibility for the use of the products described. Treatments and side effects described in this book may not be applicable to all patients; likewise, some patients may require a dose or experience a side effect that is not described herein. The reader should confer with his or her own physician regarding specific treatments and side effects. Drugs and medical devices are discussed that may have limited availability controlled by the Food and Drug Administration (FDA) for use only in a research study or clinical trial. The drug information presented has been derived from reference sources, recently published data, and pharmaceutical research data. Research, clinical practice, and government regulations often change the accepted standard in this field. When consideration is being given to use of any drug in the clinical setting, the health care provider or reader is responsible for determining FDA status of the drug, reading the package insert, reviewing prescribing information for the most up-to-date recommendations on dose, precautions, and contraindications, and determining the appropriate usage for the product. This is especially important in the case of drugs that are new or seldom used.

Production Credits
Executive Editor: Kevin Sullivan
Acquisitions Editor: Emily Ekle
Associate Editor: Amy Sibley
Editorial Assistant: Patricia Donnelly
Production Director: Amy Rose
Production Editor: Carolyn F. Rogers
Senior Marketing Manager: Katrina Gosek
Associate Marketing Manager: Rebecca Wasley
Manufacturing and Inventory Coordinator: Amy Bacus
Compositor: NK Graphics
Cover Design: Timothy Dziewit
Cover Image: © Photos.com
Printing and Binding: Courier Stoughton
Cover Printing: Courier Stoughton

Library of Congress Cataloging-in-Publication Data
AACN protocols for practice. Creating healing environments / edited by Nancy C.
  Molter.—2nd ed.
    p. ; cm.
  Includes bibliographical references.
  ISBN-13: 978-0-7637-4895-1 (pbk. : alk. paper)
  ISBN-10: 0-7637-4895-1 (pbk. : alk. paper)
  1. Intensive care nursing. 2. Family—Psychology. 3. Healing. I. Molter, Nancy C. II. Title: American Association
of Critical-Care Nurses protocols for practice. III. Title: Protocols for practice. IV. Title: Creating healing
environments.
  [DNLM: 1. Critical Care—methods. 2. Clinical Protocols. 3. Complementary Therapies—methods. 4. Critical
Illness—nursing. 5. Family—psychology. 6. Nursing Care—methods. WY 154 A1117 2007]
  RT120.15A2387 2007
  610.73'6—dc22
                                                                        2007005249

6048

Printed in the United States of America
11 10 09 08 07   10 9 8 7 6 5 4 3 2 1

Contents

About the Protocols

Recognizing that clinical practice must continually evolve to keep up with current science, busy bedside clinicians and advanced practice nurses asked the American Association of Critical-Care Nurses for help in using available research to change acute and critical care practice. They asked for studies to be translated into a format in which findings were demystified and their strength evaluated. They would use this tool to advocate for necessary changes in practice because such changes were based on the latest evidence and because they carried the weight of the association's credibility and influence.

In 1994 the American Association of Critical-Care Nurses began developing research-based practice protocols as one of several responses to this request. AACN's *Protocols for Practice* are designed to provide clinicians at the point of care with the latest patient care research findings in a format that is easy to understand and integrate into clinical practice. The protocols outline the latest thinking on how to best provide care when using technology and in specific patient care situations. Experts in each topic area develop a concise list of recommendations that are appropriate to incorporate into practice routines for patients with a particular situation or device. Recommendations are based on a comprehensive review of the science related to the situation or technology and include only those that are based on research and/or expert consensus positions.

PROTOCOL STRUCTURE

Clinical recommendations represent the core of each protocol. Recommendations are organized in a logical order, usually chronologically, starting with the time before a device is used or an occurrence begins and continuing until after the device is discontinued or the occurrence ends. Recommendations address the following:

Selection of Patients: Including indications, contraindications, and special considerations for use, such as age, physiologic status, and intermittent or continuous monitoring. Depending on the device or procedure, a clinical decision-making algorithm may be provided.

Application of Device and Initial Use: Where appropriate, important considerations during device or procedure application, such as patient preparation, preapplication calibration, and preparation of application site.

Ongoing Monitoring: Important considerations for maintaining the patient during the procedure or for monitoring the device, such as monitoring frequency and clinical factors influencing accuracy and positioning.

Prevention of Complications: Key strategies for prevention or early identification of complications, such as infection, skin breakdown, pain, or discomfort.

Quality Control: Requirements to maintain accuracy of the device under circumstances of normal use.

Recommendation Level: Each recommendation is rated according to the level of information available to support the statement. A scale ranging from I to VI represents progressively stronger levels of scientific basis for the recommendation. Ratings are defined as:

I Manufacturer's recommendation only
II Theory-based. No research data to support recommendations; recommendations from expert consensus groups may exist
III Laboratory data only, no clinical data to support recommendations
IV Limited clinical studies to support recommendations
V Clinical studies in more than 1 or 2 different populations and situations to support recommendations
VI Clinical studies in a variety of patient populations and situations to support recommendations

Along with clinical recommendations, each protocol includes these elements:

- **Case Study:** One or more brief case studies describing a common patient care situation related to the protocol topic
- **General Description:** General description of the device or patient care situation addressed by the protocol

- **Accuracy:** For medical devices, a general description of the accuracy of the device, including precision and bias, with range of accuracy given when variation exists between models and/or manufacturers
- **Competency:** Specific skill or knowledge verification that is important in determining a nurse's competency
- **Ethical Considerations:** Ethical implications or considerations related to the device or patient care situation
- **Occupational Hazards:** Hazards that may be associated with a device or patient care situation, such as electrical safety or exposure to blood-borne pathogens
- **Future Research:** Suggested areas of future research needed to strengthen the research basis of practice related to the protocol content. This may include key points of research methodology important for clinical studies in this category, such as dependent variables to be measured or confounding variables to be considered.
- **Annotated Bibliography:** Summary of important aspects of key studies on the topic
- **Suggested Readings:** Resources for additional information on the protocol topic

USING THE PROTOCOLS

The protocols are designed to guide care in a variety of acute and critical care settings, including intensive care, progressive care, and medical-surgical units. Selected topics may also be appropriate for long-term and home care. Clinicians should select those elements that apply to their practice setting.

The protocols are not intended to be used as a step-by-step procedure or comprehensive education resource alone. For this reason, each protocol includes additional information sources. Where available and appropriate, protocols include other essential information such as details about the proper application of devices or patient management algo-rithms. Clinicians may consider first using a protocol to assess the topic's current status in their practice. From this baseline assessment, they can evaluate the merits of changing current practice drawing from the protocol's evaluation of evidence that would support a change in practice.

Protocols will be valuable adjuncts in nursing education because they succinctly summarize the state of the science on a specific topic and identify areas for future research. Nursing students are often exposed to wide variation in practice in equally varied clinical settings. Protocols help to identify whether a variation is based on science.

Experienced researchers will find the protocols useful in identifying areas of inquiry. The evidence supporting each action in a protocol is rated according to its level of scientific information. Lower-level ratings indicate there is insufficient research to support a strong scientific base. Users with limited expertise in research methods will find that the protocols accurately summarize the research base using a user-friendly, concise approach with minimal jargon. They have been reviewed for scientific merit, readability, and clinical usefulness as of the time of publication.

AACN PRACTICE ALERTS

Recognizing that clinical practice is ever evolving, the American Association of Critical-Care Nurses issues practice alerts as a real-time complement to the protocols. Practice alerts are succinct dynamic directives supported by authoritative evidence to ensure excellence in practice and a safe and humane work environment. The alerts address nursing and multidisciplinary activities of importance to acutely and critically ill patients and environments in order to close the gap between research and practice, provide guidance in changing practice, standardize practice, and identify and inform about advances and new trends in the science. Practice alerts are posted at www.aacn.org.

Acknowledgments

Thanks to the scientific and clinic reviewers who assisted in developing the second edition of these protocols:

- Environmental Design and Strategies to Promote Healing—Dorrie K. Fontaine, Mary Fran Tracy
- Family Needs, Intervention, and Presence; Family Visitation and Partnership; and Family Pet Visiting and Animal-Assisted Therapy—Elizabeth A. Henneman, Joanne M. Krumberger
- Spiritual and Complementary Therapies to Promote Healing and Reduce Stress—Cathleen Guzzetta, Mary Fran Tracy
- Pain Management—Julie A. Stanik-Hutt, Evelyn F. Taverna

Special thanks to the contributors of the first edition: Marita Titler, Lynn Keegan, Julie Stanik-Hutt, Kathy Culpepper Richards, and Jane Stover Leske.

Thanks to Teresa Wavra and Ellen French of the AACN national office staff, whose assistance was invaluable to many aspects of the project.

Special appreciation goes to Marianne Chulay, who developed and implemented the practice protocols initiative for the American Association of Critical-Care Nurses.

The author thanks the Family Intervention Research Team at The University of Iowa Hospitals and Clinics for their conduct and use of research for families of critically ill patients.

Contributors

Richard B. Arbour, RN, MSN, CCRN, CNRN
Staff Nurse
Albert Einstein Healthcare Net
Philadelphia, Pennsylvania

Jane Stover Leske, RN, PhD
Associate Professor
College of Nursing
University of Wisconsin-Milwaukee
Milwaukee, Wisconsin

Nancy C. Molter, RN, MN, PhD
Choctaw Management Services Enterprises
Clinical Research Coordinator Program Manager
US Army Institute of Surgical Research
Fort Sam Houston, Texas

Mae Ann Pasquale, RN, MSN, CCRN
Assistant Professor
Cedar Crest College
Allentown, Pennsylvania

Monica A. Redekopp, MN, RN
Director, Professional Nursing Practice
Crouse Hospital
Syracuse, New York

Stephanie Woods, RN, PhD
Consultant
San Antonio, Texas

Environmental Design and Strategies to Promote Healing

Nancy C. Molter, RN, MN, PhD

Environmental Design and Strategies to Promote Healing

CASE STUDY

The Beginning

Jim, a candidate for acute and critical care director, walked into the surgical Intensive Care Unit (ICU) for the first time after noticing the large sign explaining that visiting hours were 10 minutes an hour from 10 AM to 12 PM and from 4 PM to 7 PM. He stood quietly and observed the area. The lights were bright and glaring on the plain, cream-colored walls. There was an abstract geometric designed wallpaper border along the tops of the walls but no other art work in the area. Ten single-patient rooms encircled a central nursing station. Each room was enclosed with wide glass doors fronting the room. Each room had a window, although the rooms along the east wall faced an inner courtyard surrounded on all 4 sides by hospital walls. Sunlight was abundant, but the view out the window was to a cement courtyard with a few scattered benches. Privacy curtains, matching the wallpaper border along the ceiling, could be pulled over the room doors. Furniture in the rooms consisted of a bed, night stand, and bed tray. A few rooms had a cardiac chair for patient use. A clock was on the wall facing each bed. Jim noticed the loud sounds coming from the equipment and staff conversations. There was a separate entrance from the unit to the operating room suite. He liked the location of the progressive care unit in relation to the ICU. It was just out the front doors and across a hallway that passed by the family waiting room.

The staff lounge was small and located just off the entrance to the ICU. It contained a small table, some lockers, a wall-mounted cubby hole unit for staff mail, a wall-mounted TV, and a refrigerator. Bulletin boards held hospital notices. He also noted that the family waiting room was just off the ICU, and the entrance was monitored by a hospital volunteer. There was a small, separate room for family consultations. Furniture consisted of industrial waiting room couches, a few arm chairs, two coffee tables, and a counter containing a coffee pot and supplies. There was one telephone available in the open area.

In speaking with the hospital administration and unit staff members, Jim understood that renovations were going to be made. Staffing appeared adequate but turnover was high. Support service personnel such as chaplains, social workers, case managers, and the clinical nurse specialist were interested in complementary therapies but were unsure how to introduce them into the unit. Administration was interested in the philosophy of patient/family-centered care and creating healing environments. Physicians were noncommittal about the concept.

As Jim absorbed the environment, he made the decision that the elements were favorable in the organization for a culture change to create a healing environment. When offered the management position, he accepted.

Two Years Later

It was 6 AM and Jim was in the surgical ICU for a staff meeting with the night shift. He reflected on how quiet the unit was and that lighting was conducive to promoting sleep. The warm serene colors of the walls were complementary to the full spectrum colors reflected in the pastoral and floral art work present in each patient's room and in the staff and family lounges. He stopped into Mrs J's room. She was successfully being weaned from the ventilator after being on it for 3 weeks. Mrs J was awake and listening to music as she prepared for her next weaning session. She indicated that she had a good night's sleep without interruption since 10 PM. She was looking forward to the sunrise so that she could see the beautiful garden outside her window in the hospital atrium. The fresh scent of lavender filled her room from the essential oil that was brought in by her daughter.

As Jim entered the staff lounge, he smiled at the newest bulletin board decoration. Each staff member brought in a baby picture and there was a contest to see who could identify the most pictures. He read the latest thank-you note from a grateful patient and family also posted on the "Chicken Soup for the Nurses' Soul" board. He noted that families appreciated the pictures of the staff posted on the wall as they entered the unit. It helped them identify who was caring for their significant other. Although this family had just lost their father, they were grateful that they were present during the resuscitation efforts and could be with him as he passed away. Jim was particularly pleased that the "Visitor Regulations" sign at the entrance to the unit was removed. The patient/family needs for presence in the unit were addressed individually rather than with a blanket visiting policy.

As Jim sank into the comfortable chair in the staff lounge, he reflected on today's agenda. With the decrease in staff turnover, there was time and enthusiasm among staff to help with developing policies. Two policies were to be discussed. One was pet visitation and animal-assisted activities. There were increased requests for such visits, and the physicians and infection control nurse were concerned about infections. The other policy related to family presence during resuscitation and invasive procedures. A final draft was being presented for staff approval. Using the AACN Practice Alerts and Healing Environment protocols greatly assisted in the development of these policies.

Jim was proud of the achievements of the staff and administration in creating a healing environment over the past 2 years. He looked forward to the Healing Environment group meeting this afternoon composed of community members, past patients and families, and clinicians to set the agenda for future activities to create a healing environment for all. This group developed the blueprint for the physical and administrative changes that had already been made. The members looked forward to continued integration of environmental strategies to promote healing.

GENERAL DESCRIPTION

Creating a humane and healing environment for acute and critical care requires a systemic approach to designing health care delivery systems. "*Healing* is the dynamic process of recovery, repair, restoration, renewal, and transformation that increases resilience, coherence, and wholeness (Suggested Readings: 10, p 38)." "An *optimal healing environment* is a system and place composed of people, behaviors, treatments, and their psychological and physical parameters. Its purpose is to provide conditions that stimulate and support the inherent healing capacities of the participants, their relationships, and their surroundings (Suggested Readings: 10, p. 38)." Jonas et al (Suggested Readings: 10) propose that these definitions be used in future research, along with those listed in Table 1-1, to facilitate consistent communication

relative to defining an optimal healing environment. In the 2001 Institute of Medicine report, *Crossing the Quality Chasm: A New Health System for the 21st Century*, healing is stated as a core mission of health care in general (Suggested Readings: 9). A new investment of research in healing is needed.

There is a science related to healing processes called *salutogenesis*; this term describes the processes of healing that strive toward human growth and development. There is a need to expand the research base of conventional, complementary, and alternative therapies to promote healing (Suggested Readings: 10, 11). What models for synergistic healing exist? Is there an economic value to caring? What evidence exists that organizational cultures of healing are effective?

Theoretical/Philosophical Foundation for Healing Environments

The concept of the environment contributing to healing is not new. In ancient cultures, manipulating the environment to place the body in the best position to heal itself was often the only strategy available. There are 2 models to explore in creating healing environments today: cultural and organizational models.

Cultural Models

There is a rich history of healing models from several cultures. The ancient medicine of Indian cultures, Ayurveda, describes access to a universal consciousness through meditation and intention that restores order and health to persons and communities. The traditional Chinese medicine considers "qi" the life energy responsible for health, illness, and healing. American Indians used specific rituals and altered states of consciousness to manipulate spiritual forces thought to be the cause of illness (Suggested Readings: 10). However, in the United States, alternative forms of medicine have been marginalized in the health care system. Despite their widespread use, "energy"-based practices are viewed with skepticism. Fortunately, there is a National Institute of Health Center for Complementary and Alternative Medicine (NCCAM) with a mission to explore the science of such practices (http://nccam.nih.gov).

To create healing environments there must be an organizational philosophy and commitment to structuring the resources to support the philosophy and to focus on integrating science and spirituality. Malloch (Annotated Bibliography: 2) lists 5 common components of organizational healing models:

1. Common values of health as a function of body-mind-spirit interrelationships
2. Patient-centered relationships
3. An organizational culture that supports personal growth and mastery
4. The availability of alternative therapies in addition to conventional health care therapies
5. A physical environment that supports healing

Table 1-1   Proposed Definitions for Use in Research Related to Optimal Healing Environment

Healing	The dynamic process of recovery, repair, restoration, renewal, and transformation that increases resilience, coherence, and wholeness. An emergent process of the person's whole system (physical, mental, social, spiritual, and environmental). It may or may not involve curing.
Optimal healing environment	A system and place composed of people, behaviors, treatments, and their psychological and physical parameters. Its purpose is to provide conditions that stimulate and support the inherent healing capacities of the participants, their relationships, and their surroundings. May include general and specific physical, behavioral, psychological, social, and spiritual components including medical treatment.
Healing intention and awareness	The mindful determination by one or more participants through both intuitive and conscious action to improve the health of another person or oneself. Uses intention and education to increase awareness of, and then to establish, hope, belief, and expectation in the possibility of wholeness, well-being, and positive change.
Healing presence and energy	A deep presence that enhances recovery and repair. A physical and emotional wholeness from which deep personal engagement, caring, and communication emerge. In Eastern cultures this presence is often expressed as "bioenergy" and is believed to be accumulated, stored, and transmitted between healer and healee.
Healing relationships	Consist of 2 domains that involve the designated clinician or others: (1) therapeutic alliance, or the relationship that encompasses the embodied social and psychological interactions between healers and healee that facilitate healing; and (2) the domain that involves social and community relationships. Characteristics of both domains include empathy, compassion, beneficence, mindfulness, demeanor, caring, hope, love, inspiration, reassurance, comfort, warmth, trust, confidence, credibility, honesty, expectation, courtesy, respect, harmony, challenge, and communication.
Health-promoting behavior	The employment of adequate amounts and types of exercise, diet, relaxation, creative outlets, social service and support, and spiritual development.
Healing collaborations	These arise from healing relationships for the purpose of identification, choice, and application of individualized treatments and care strategies. Selection of treatment is a combination of science, experience, and values and requires a dynamic and trusting interaction to identify the best treatment for individual situations.
Healing treatments	Methods to stimulate the body's healing processes and repair with a focus on disease management and goal of cure when appropriate. Includes conventional medical therapies and complementary and alternative therapies.
Healing spaces	The physical environment, including the visual esthetics, sound, music, smell, taste, lighting, air, art, water, horticulture, architecture, and conditioning processes that support and stimulate recovery and repair processes.

Source: Jonas WB, Chez R, Duffy B. Investigating the impact of optimal healing environments. *Alternative Ther.* 2003;9(6):36-40.

These components, when integrated with cultural sensitivity, can greatly improve the healing aspects of the health care environment. Unfortunately there is little evidence of organizational healing models and their effects on patient outcomes. However, a few models are reported in the literature as described in the next section.

Organizational Healing Models

Organizational healing models require a multidisciplinary team approach to achieve desired outcomes (Annotated Bibliography: 1-4; Suggested Readings: 3, 8, 16: Other References: 1, 2, 4, 8, 10, 11, 14). Patients tell us that communication among team members is often remembered and that it can continue to affect the patient even after discharge (Annotated Bibliography: 1; Suggested Readings: 13). Several studies specific to the critical care environment demonstrated that physician-nurse collaboration was a significant factor in decreasing predicted mortality and morbidity, decreasing staff turnover, and increasing patient and staff satisfaction with care (Other References: 1, 8, 10, 11).

Nursing presence is also a key element to the patient's outcome (Suggested Readings: 4-6; Other References 10, 11). There are 6 features of nursing presence that compose the context of nursing judgment (Suggested Readings: 6): uniqueness; connecting with the patient's experience, sensing; going beyond scientific data; knowing what will work and when to act; and being with the patient. The essence of nursing presence is embodied in the American Association of Critical-Care Nurses Synergy Model for Patient Care (Annotated Bibliography: 4; Suggested Readings: 2, 5, 7).

The AACN Synergy Model for Patient Care

The AACN Synergy Model for Patient Care was developed to conceptualize certified critical care nursing practice as recognizing that the needs and characteristics of patients and families influence and drive the competencies of nurses. The model evolved from the AACN vision of a health care system driven by the needs of patients and families in which critical care nurses can make their optimal contributions. The basic assumptions of the model are (Suggested Readings: 2, 5):

- That all patients are biological, psychological, social, and spiritual entities with similar needs and experiences at any particular developmental stage over a continuum of health and illness.
- The dimensions of a nurse's practice can be described along continua and are determined by the patient and family needs.
- The context of the nurse-patient relationship is based on contributions from the patient, family, and community.
- Optimal outcomes can be achieved with the synergy that develops through the alignment of nurse competencies with patient/family needs.

The model describes 8 characteristics of patients that drive 8 characteristics of nurses' practice to meet those needs. Optimal outcomes for the patient/family, nurse practice, and health care organization are based on the synergy that develops when care is provided based on this model (Suggested Readings: 2, 5). This model incorporates the therapeutic use of the nurse's presence to facilitate healing. In a comprehensive study, the model was validated for critical care nursing practice (Annotated Bibliography: 4). Patient characteristics are defined as follows (the first 5 being intrinsic to the patient and the last 3 extrinsic and related to environment and resources):

- Resiliency—The capacity to return to a restorative level of functioning using compensatory or coping mechanisms; the ability to bounce back after an insult
- Vulnerability—Susceptibility to actual or potential stressors that may adversely affect patient outcomes
- Stability—The ability to maintain a steady-state equilibrium
- Complexity—The intricate entanglement of 2 or more systems (eg, boy, family, therapies)
- Predictability—A characteristics that allows one to expect a certain course of events or course of illness
- Resource availability—Extent of resources (eg, technical, fiscal, personal, psychological, and social) that the patient/family/community brings to the situation
- Participation in care—Extent to which patient and family engages in aspects of care
- Participation in decision making—Extent to which patient and family engages in decision making

The following 8 nursing characteristics range from a competent to expert level:

- Clinical judgment—Clinical reasoning, which includes clinical decision making, critical thinking, and a global grasp of the situation, coupled with nursing skills acquired through a process of integrating formal and experiential knowledge.
- Advocacy/moral agency—Working on another's behalf and representing the concerns of the patient, family, and community; serving as a moral agent in identifying and helping to resolve ethical and clinical concerns within the clinical setting.

- Caring practices—The constellation of nursing activities that are responsive to the uniqueness of the patient and family and that create a compassionate and therapeutic environment, with the aim of promoting comfort and preventing suffering. These caring behaviors include, but are not limited to, vigilance, engagement, and responsiveness.
- Collaboration—Working with others (eg, patients, families, health care providers) in a way that promotes and encourages each person's contributions toward achieving optimal and realistic patient goals. Collaboration involves intra- and interdisciplinary work with all colleagues.
- Systems thinking—The body of knowledge and tools that allow the nurse to appreciate the care environment from a perspective that recognizes the holistic interrelationship that exists within and across health care systems.
- Response to diversity—The sensitivity to recognize, appreciate, and incorporate differences into the provision of care. Differences may include, but are not limited to, individuality, cultural differences (eg, in child rearing, family relations), spiritual beliefs, gender, race, ethnicity, disability, family configuration, lifestyle, socioeconomic status, age values, and alternative medicine involving patients and their families and members of the health care team.
- Clinical inquiry or Innovator/evaluator—The ongoing process of questioning and evaluating practice, providing informed practice, and innovating through research and experiential learning. The nurse engages in clinical knowledge development to promote the best patient outcomes.
- Facilitator of learning or patient/family educator—The ability to facilitate patient and family learning.

The environment has particular significance within the Synergy Model because of the reciprocal relationship between the nurse and the environment (Suggested Readings: 7). The nature of this reciprocal relationship may be influenced by factors such as the setting, the particular situation, and the nurse's experience. Although nurses create the immediate environment at the point of care, the environment can influence what the nurse is and is not able to do. Therefore, the environment can influence the extent and quality of the synergy that occurs between the nurse and the patient. That synergy can, in turn, have an effect on the environment.

Optimal outcomes are achieved when the patient characteristics influence and drive the required level of nursing competency. Three types of outcomes are depicted in the Synergy Model:

- Patient outcomes—Behavior change based on dispensing or receiving information; measured with functional and quality-of-life measurements, satisfaction ratings, and comfort ratings and perceptions.
- Nurse-derived outcomes—Includes physiologic changes, the presence or absence of preventable complications,

and the extent to which care and treatment objectives are attained.

- System outcomes—Recidivism and cost/resource utilization: Resource utilization incorporates nurse turnover. Nurses leave environments where they cannot function in an optimal manner to achieve positive patient outcomes.

There are no specific outcome studies using the Synergy Model; however, a clinical demonstration project is underway at Clarian Health Partners to implement this model across the 1200-bed health system's three main campuses in Indianapolis, Ind. (http://www.clarian.org/clarianjobs/nursing/synergy.htm). As well, Duquesne University School of Nursing in Pittsburgh, Pa, has adopted the model as the basis for its undergraduate and graduate curricula. (http://www.nursingknowledge.org/Portal/main.aspx?pageid=3507&ContentID=56395)

The AACN Certification Corporation Web site has continuous updates on articles that link the model to a variety of practice environments (http://www.certcorp.org).

The Healthy Organization Model
This model was developed from Malloch's study that explored 3 of the 5 organizational components that form a framework for creating a healing organizational environment (Annotated Bibliography: 2). The 3 components studied included:

1. Common values of health as a function of body-mind-spirit interrelationships. Two characteristics defined this component: an orientation to wellness, and congruence between individual and organizational perspectives. The orientation to wellness is defined by health values focused on adaptive ability, role function, self-actualization, and being loved. Illness-related clinical health values are valued but are considered incomplete in defining health values. To achieve congruence between individual and organizational perspectives of common values of health, all stakeholders (eg, caregivers, consumers, and community members) must value holistic health.
2. Patient-centered relationships are the basis of all patient activities. The patients' personal values are respected and health care decisions are based on the patient's beliefs, values, and choices. In the organization, patient centeredness is reflected in continuity of services, grouping of patients based on common needs, and responsive services. Patient-centered care is well defined by the landmark study completed by the Picker/Commonwealth Program for Patient-Centered Care (Annotated Bibliography: 1). In a national survey of patients and their families, 7 dimensions were identified that are viewed as important to patients and families "through the patient's eyes":

- Respect for patients' values, preference, and expressed needs
- Coordination and integration of care
- Information, communication, and education
- Physical discomfort
- Emotional support and alleviation of fear and anxiety
- Involvement of family and friends
- Transition and continuity

3. An organizational culture that supports growth and personal mastery promotes lifelong learning and facilitates the organization's survival through the development of capacity in their human capital. An essential measure of this component is job satisfaction. In Malloch's study 5 characteristics were evaluated in relation to job satisfaction (Annotated Bibliography: 2): supervisor support; clarity of expectations in terms of knowing what is expected in the role and how explicitly rules and policies are communicated; involvement of employees; peer cohesion; and innovation as reflected by degree of emphasis on variety and change and an autonomous practice environment. This was one of the first organizational models examined that indicated an economic value to holistic care.

The Planetree Model
Planetree is a holistic care model developed in 1978 by a patient, Angelica Thieriot. She experienced several traumatic hospitalizations where the technical care was fine but she felt depersonalized by the experience. A 13-bed medical/surgical unit in San Francisco became the first Planetree unit in the country. There are now more than 80 health care centers in the United States and Canada that use this patient-centered model. There are 9 elements in the Planetree model (Annotated Bibliography: 3; Other References: 14):

1. Human interactions should be about people caring about other people. This includes how patients are cared for, how staff care for themselves and each other, and how organizations create a culture that supports and nurtures their staff. Healing partnerships are created between patients, family members, and caregivers.
2. Empowering patients through information and education is implemented through programs that customize information and education packets, hold collaborative care conferences, and develop collaborative patient pathways. There is an open chart policy to promote trust and help patients and families learn about their health care. Information is available to the community through resource libraries.
3. The importance of family, friends, and social support networks is acknowledged. The Care Partner Program provides training to assist family members to participate in care. There is unrestricted visiting hours, even in the ICU.
4. Spirituality is facilitated in the Planetree model. There are chapels, meditation rooms, and gardens to provide opportunities for prayer and reflection. Chaplains are a vital member of the team.
5. Human touch is an essential way of communication. Therapeutic massage is available for patients, family, and staff.

6. Arts and entertainment are viewed as nutrition for the soul. Artists and musicians are involved in helping patients. Music, storytellers, clowns, and funny movies are available.

7. Complementary therapies are incorporated into care. Aromatherapy, pet therapy, mind-body-spirit medicine interventions are all being used with increasing frequency.

8. Architectural and interior design conducive to health and healing are incorporated in the home-like environments and the provision for space, privacy, and dignity.

9. Nutrition is recognized as an integral part of health. Healthy food choices are emphasized in the dining rooms and vending machines. Kitchens are available on the patient care floors to assist families in preparing food for their loved ones. They also become informal support centers for family members.

Without an underlying philosophical commitment and organizational structure to integrate all the necessary elements of a healing environment, true progress will not be achieved. The environment must be healing for the staff as well as the patients and families. The physical environment in staff lounges should provide an oasis to help reduce stress during a shift. Staff policies need to address the importance of humane scheduling, reduction of verbal and physical violence (http://www.aacn.org for fact sheets and position statements on these issues), and the need to develop competency in negotiating skills and conflict management (Suggested Readings: 8, 12; Other References: 1, 9, 13). With an organizational structure in place that integrates all components of a healing environment, the physical environment can be adapted or constructed to promote healing. Such a physical environment includes space and design elements to promote safety and comfort; prevent hospital-acquired infections; and promote sleep and relaxation through noise reduction, use of music, and therapeutic use of aroma, light, and color.

COMPETENCY

Knowledge of the use of complementary therapies requires study and practice. In addition, there must be an organizational culture that facilitates use of complementary and alternative therapies to conventional medical practices to create true healing practices. It requires a team of people (administrators, architects, engineers, clinicians, consumers) to create an environment that contributes to healing. No one stakeholder group can do it alone (Suggested Readings: 8; Other References: 15). Team work requires skills in negotiation and conflict management (Other References: 9). To that end, acute and critical care nurses must be knowledgeable of the value of contributions of others and be actively involved in designing an integrated system for healing. In 2005, the American Association of Critical-Care Nurses published a set of *essential* standards for establishing and sustaining healthy work environments (Suggested Readings: 1).

They are considered essential because of the increasing body of evidence that unhealthy work environments contribute to medical errors, increased staff stress and anxiety, and ineffective and poor quality of care. The 6 standards are:

- Nurses must be as proficient in communication skills as they are in clinical skills.
- Nurses must be relentless in pursuing and fostering true collaboration.
- Nurses must be valued and committed partners in making policy, directing and evaluating clinical care, and leading organizational operations.
- Staffing must ensure the effective match between patient needs and nurse competencies.
- Nurses must be recognized and must recognize others for the value each brings to the work of the organization.
- Nurse leaders must fully embrace the imperative of a healthy work environment, authentically live it, and engage others in its achievement.

Developing competency in practice involves managing the physical environment to promote healing and safety. Providing complex care requires skills in system thinking, clinical judgment, inquiry, and caring practices to create the right environment for a specific patient. Knowledge of research-based practices is essential for this type of expert care. All nurses need to be familiar with the environment of care standards set by the Joint Commission on Accreditation of Healthcare Organizations and the Centers for Disease Control and Prevention for the prevention of infections (Suggested Readings: 24; Other References: 18), as well as the AACN Standards for Establishing and Sustaining Healthy Work Environments (Suggested Readings: 1).

ETHICAL CONSIDERATIONS

Humane care means caring for the acute and critically ill patient as a whole person and as a member of a family and community. The principles of autonomy and beneficence are integral to humane care. Is it ethical to enforce separation of the patient from the rest of the family unnecessarily, especially at the time of death? Is it ethical to care for a patient in an environment that is not safe, that could lead to life-threatening infections or even hearing disorders due to environmental noise? Is it ethical to induce delirium due to lack of sleep? Is it ethical to treat depression with just medications and not consider therapeutic use of light or pet-assisted therapies? Providing humane care mandates that we use the environment as a tool for healing.

SUMMARY OF CURRENT RESEARCH ABOUT HEALING ENVIRONMENTS

The human being assesses the environment through 5 senses: sight, hearing, touch, smell, and taste. Therefore, the modification of the environment should address these senses. It is important to consider stimuli that affect the senses in relation to the science of chronobiology, or the study of biologic rhythms. Biologic rhythms in human beings are generated from within the organism but can be affected by environmental stimuli in the critical care unit (Suggested Readings: 15; Other References: 77). There are 2 effects: transient, such as occurs when a patient reacts to a sudden noise or heart rate increases during painful procedures; and entrainment, that occurs when the biological rhythms are synchronized to patterns of environmental stimuli (Suggested Readings: 15, 31). Examples are the rhythms of temperature control, light-dark cycles, and patterns of social cues (Suggested Readings: 15). These patterns will resynchronize to the environment over time. However, many patients in the ICU do not stay long enough for the resynchronization to occur. Thus sleep is often affected and discomfort is perceived more acutely due to environmental temperature. This internal desynchronization may impair functioning and exacerbate critical illness (Suggested Readings: 15, 31). The impact of the environment has greater affect on the patient who cannot leave or control their environment (Suggested Readings: 5, 14, 15: Other References: 3, 7, 21, 22).

Sight

The complementary therapies related to visual stimulation include light therapy and the effects of color and art.

Light is needed for physical and psychological well-being. Using light to heal is an ancient therapy. One of the key considerations of light in the critical care unit is the use of full versus incomplete spectrum of lighting. Color is derived from light; it is our perception of light of different wavelengths. Increased levels of ACTH and cortisol (the stress hormones) have been measured in individuals sitting under cool-white lighting provided by most florescent lights. Based on initial studies of such lighting, cool-white fluorescent bulbs are banned from German hospital and medical facilities (Suggested Readings: 16, 21, 22, 31).

The pineal gland regulates the onset of puberty, induces sleep, and influences our moods. It also acts as the body's light meter and timer by synchronizing with the external environment. Artificial light artificially manipulates the pineal gland's functions. Melatonin is the hormone produced by the pineal gland that influences sleep. Melatonin is normally highest at nighttime, but the level can be reduced by artificial light (Suggested Readings: 16, 31). Therefore, the type of lighting and the use of lighting appear to have a significant role in creating a healing environment in acute care.

Color has been shown to affect feelings and emotions, as well as mood, breathing rate, pulse rate, and blood pressure (Suggested Readings: 14, 31, 32; Other References: 74, 75, 78, 79). Early research indicated that blue, green, and black decrease blood pressure, heart rate, and respiratory rate, while warmer colors such as red, orange, and yellow simulate the body. Studies today continue to indicate that colors

affect our moods and physiologic responses in the same manner. Using a balance of colors in hospital rooms tends to create a balance in emotions.

Art can create moods in 4 ways: the specific colors used, the subject matter, the size of the art, and the style of art (Other References: 71; Suggested Readings 28). In a study involving open-heart surgery patients exposed to art with a nature theme versus abstract art, it was clear that the nature themes were more soothing to patients and reduced their anxiety and pain (Annotated Bibliography: 10). Cohen described a process to assist hospital committees charged with selecting art to choose the most appropriate art that is likely to promote a sense of well-being (Other References: 70).

Light, color, and nature do heal. Ulrich first showed the effect of having a window in a patient's room on healing (Other References: 76). Today, all patients in a hospital are required to have a "room with a view" (Other References: 18). A window is not only important to bring in sunlight and maintain normal rhythmic cycles, but it should provide a view that is aesthetically pleasing. Many hospitals are providing garden views to promote calmness and reduce anxiety (Other References: 71).

Hearing

Noise produces some of the most detrimental affects on healing in hospitals and particularly in critical care units (Other References: 29. 50; Suggested Readings: 25). The Environmental Protection Agency (EPA) established guidelines for upper limits of noise in a hospital to be 45 dB during the day and 35 dB at night (Other References: 15, 16). Most studies measuring noise indicate that these levels are consistently and greatly exceeded (Suggested Readings: 25). This becomes an issue of safety as well as delayed healing (Other References: 46, 49, 61). Not only is there a significant chance of hearing loss, but there is some evidence relating increased noise to increased lengths of stay and to symptoms of stress in critical care nurses (Suggested Readings: 25). In the study by Tsiou et al, the dropping of metallic objects rated the highest (75-92 dB), and the respirators registered the lowest (49-72 dB) (Other References: 64). Cabrera and colleagues (Suggested Readings: 25) recommend the development of a department of sound to address strategies to reduce the noise in hospitals.

Music, however, can mediate the stress of noise (Other References: 39). In a comprehensive review of the literature about the effects of music on patient outcomes, music did decrease anxiety during routine care, but appears to have little effect on anxiety due to procedures (Suggested Readings: 25; Other References: 32). It has the greatest impact on reducing heart rate. Music or soothing sound is effective in increasing the mood of patients and their tolerance to care provided (Annotated Bibliography: 12; Other References: 32-39, 41, 43-45, 47-49, 51, 52, 56, 67-70).

Touch

The sense of touch includes the body's response to energy that surrounds it. Forms of touch therapy such as massage and therapeutic massage will be addressed in a separate protocol. Touching in general may be viewed as a nurturing connection if it is done with the intent to reduce anxiety and convey comfort. It is often a tangible sign of the nurse's being present with the patient (Suggested Readings: 4, 13; Other References: 8).

Although not specifically addressed in this protocol, it is also important to evaluate how the environment affects the patient's sense of feeling. Are they too warm or too cold? What is the pressure and/or thermal effect of equipment and supplies on the patient's skin? Do they need to be turned to relieve pressure points? Is furniture arranged to facilitate the need to touch for support and safety when walking in the room?

Another aspect of the sense of touch is the potential for transmission of infections through touching. The environment needs to be cleaned according to industry standards, and the staff must adhere to washing their hands before patient contact to reduce infections (Suggested Readings: 23, 24; Other References: 18, 28).

Smell

Aromatherapy is the use of essential oils to stimulate body responses via the sense of smell. To date there have been no credible studies indicating the effectiveness of such therapy in acute care. Four recent randomized trials (one double-blinded) did not demonstrate any significant results (Other References: 81-84). Though the use of essential oils may promote a sense of well-being in some patients (Other References: 81), there is the potential for reactions to the oils in acute and critically ill patients that limit their use in this environment (Other References: 80). Their use should be evaluated carefully on a case-by-case basis.

Patients can also be compromised through poor control of the quality of air in the environment. Breathing in bacteria or fumes from noxious chemicals can lead to harm. The hospital must ensure that the patient's environment has the appropriate air quality control measures to prevent secondary infection or injury (Suggested Readings: 23, 24).

Taste

There are no known complementary therapies related to the sense of taste. However, taste plays a major role in the nutritional intake of patients. Therefore, a healing environment will ensure that nutrition is carefully assessed and maintained to promote healing. When possible, the patients should be given food that they like and that stimulates appetite. The sense of taste should also be assessed in terms of its usefulness in detecting side effects of medications.

The Synergy of a Healing Environment

The effect of the environment and use of alternative or complementary forms of healing can be synergistic with the application of traditional medical science. Creating healing spaces requires an organizational commitment and willingness to explore the care delivery processes in place. Table 1-2 outlines 6 questions that organizations should answer when considering an organizational commitment to creating a healing environment (Other References: 5).

The Center for Health Design believes that investing time and capital into creating healing designs will contribute positive financial success through the following:

- Decreased lengths of stay
- Decreased costs per inpatient day as a result of decreased nursing care hours and reduced supply costs
- Decreased use of stronger pain medication
- Decreased costs through reduction in falls, nosocomial infections, and medical errors
- Increased staff and physician satisfaction and retention
- Increased market share due to patient satisfaction (Other References: 5)

The current challenge is to measure such outcomes. For example, in an extensive review of the literature concerning the impact of hospital architecture on the development of nosocomial infections, there was a lack of evidence of a direct connection due to the multifactoral nature of nosocomial infections (Annotated Bibliography: 6). On the other hand, measuring the impact of acuity-adaptable unit designs that decrease the movement of patients in the hospital demonstrates safety implications of reduced medical errors and injuries and labor cost saving (Suggested Readings: 14; Other References: 23).

Clinically, many of the aspects of a healing environment are embodied in strategies to reduce pain and anxiety and to promote relaxation and sleep. Separate protocols in this series will address the reduction of pain and anxiety, the inclusion of family-centered care principals to reduce anxiety, and the use of strategies to produce relaxation. This protocol will specifically address strategies to promote sleep.

Table 1-2   Organizational Assessment of Commitment to a Healing Environment Philosophy

1. What are the core elements that define your hospital's cultural understanding of healing environments?

2. Do your care delivery processes support the healing environment?

3. What do your patients and their families say are important elements of a healing environment?

4. What specifically are the top priorities for creating healing spaces?

5. How many of your goals can be accomplished with change in care delivery and service versus remodeling the facilities?

6. Are you also prepared to commit the operational dollars to orient staff and physicians to the care philosophy of healing environments, and train them to provide the care and service to fully optimize the new environment?

Source: Goe, SJ. Beyond waterfalls and grand pianos. *Healthcare Exec.* 2003;18(4):68-69.

Promotion of Sleep

This protocol will focus only on environmental strategies to promote sleep. However, pharmacologic interventions to reduce pain and anxiety and thus promote sleep should be considered for all acute and critically ill patients. Sleep disturbances involve inability to fall asleep, maintain sleep, or early awakening (Suggested Readings: 30). Acute and critically ill patients experience all these disturbances due to environment conditions. Lighting, noise, and hospital and treatment routines are constant challenges to developing sleep hygiene protocols to assist patients to have healing sleep periods (Annotated Bibliography: 7; Suggested Readings: 26-28; Other References: 29, 46-50, 51, 55, 59). The nurse needs to assess these factors to develop a plan for promoting sleep for individual patients (Annotated Bibliography: 9; Suggested Readings: 25-27; Other References 57-59, 62). The hospital needs to evaluate general environmental conditions that contribute to reducing sleep and design strategies to control these factors. Such strategies include the use of acoustic tile and floor materials that reduce noise; policies related to use of overhead paging and use of call systems in all rooms to seek staff and make announcements; lighting sources and use of light to induce normal light-dark cycles; and the use of music and other relaxing sounds to mitigate background noise and promote relaxation (Other References: 57, 58; Suggested Readings: 25, 29). Background noise in hospitals can be caustic and harmful to patients and staff. Strategies need to be developed that encourage staff to be more aware of reducing noise when possible from conversations and equipment (Annotated Bibliography: 7; Other References: 50, 65).

FUTURE RESEARCH

Future research on environments of healing might include the following issues or address the questions in the following sections.

Organizational Models for Healing

- Is there a valid and reliable organizational assessment tool to ascertain commitment to a healing organization philosophy?
- Are healing environments cost-effective, and what specific organizational outcomes of a healing environment can be measured reliably and validly?
- What organizational models facilitate clinical team collaboration and communication? Does an open versus closed ICU make a difference?
- Does practice based on the AACN Synergy Model affect patient and organizational outcomes?
- How does an organizational model for healing affect specific organizational outcomes?
- What impact does integrating the AACN Standards for Establishing and Sustaining Healthy Work Environments have on decreasing medical errors, decreasing staff stress

and turnover, and increasing the quality indicators of care provided?

Environmental Strategies to Promote Healing

Design

- How does hospital room design contribute to healing from the patient/family's perspective?
- Conduct randomized trials on the use of full-spectrum lighting to facilitate healing in critical care units.
- What effect does acuity-based room designs have on patient outcomes and organizational outcomes?
- How does a healing environment for staff break rooms affect staff productivity?

Infection Control

- What environmental factors contribute to effective hand washing?
- How do the use of personal equipment like stethoscopes, pagers, cell phones, and scrub attire affect infection control in the hospital? How should policies change to reflect findings?

Use of Color and Art

- Conduct more randomized trials on the use of art to facilitate relaxation.
- Is the choice of art in a patient's room an effective and feasible strategy to promote relaxation and healing in an acute care environment?

Music

- Conduct more multicentered randomized trials using music therapy protocols to reduce the pain of painful procedures.
- What is the most effective protocol for music intervention to promote relaxation in the acute and critical care environment?

Sleep Hygiene

- Is a "department of noise" concept successful in integrating noise-reducing processes in hospitals?
- What are effective environmental strategies to ensure adequate periods of sleep for acute and critically ill patients?
- How can staff be sensitized to reduce unnecessary noise and light in the acute and critical care environment?
- Are unit-based sleep hygiene protocols effective?

SUGGESTED READINGS
ORGANIZATIONAL CULTURE
OF HEALING

1. American Association of Critical Care-Nurses. *AACN Standards for Establishing and Sustaining Healthy Work Environments*. Aliso Viejo, Calf: AACN; 2003.

2. American Association of Critical-Care Nurses. The Synergy Model for Patient Care. Available at: http://www.certcorp.org/certcorp/certcorp.nsf/vwdoc/SynModel?opendocument. Accessed October 19, 2006.

3. Byers JF. Holistic acute care units: partnerships to meet the needs of the chronically ill and their families. *AACN Clin Issues*. 1997;8(2):272-279.

4. Burfitt SN, Greiner DS, Miers LJ, et al. Professional nurse caring as perceived by the critically ill patients: a phenomenologic study. *Am J Crit Care*. 1993;2(6):489-499.

5. Curley MAQ. Patient-nurse synergy: optimizing patient outcomes. *Am J of Crit Care*. 1998;7(1):64-72.

6. Doona ME, Chase SK, Haggerty LA. Nursing presence. As real as a Milky Way bar. *J Holis Nurs*. 1999;17(1):54-70.

7. Hardin SR, Kaplow R. *Synergy for Clinical Excellence: The AACN Synergy Model for Patient Care*. Sudbury Mass: Jones and Bartlett; 2005.

8. Harvey MA, Ninos, NP, Adler DC, et al. Results of the consensus conference on fostering more humane critical care: creating a healing environment. *AACN Clin Issues*. 1993;4(3):484-549.

9. Institute of Medicine. *Crossing the Quality Chasm: A New Health System for the 21st Century*. Washington DC: National Academy of Sciences Press, 2001.

10. Jonas WB, Chez, RA, Duffy B, et al. Investigating the impact of optimal healing environments. *Alt Therapies*. 2003;9(6):36-40.

11. Kligler B. Creating the optimal environment. *Alt Therapies*. 2003;9(6):34-35.

12. Molter NC. Creating a healing environment for critical care. *Crit Care Nurs Clin N Am*. 2003;15:295-304.

13. Russell S. An exploratory study of patients' perceptions, memories and experiences of an intensive care unit. *J Adv Nurs*. 1999;29(4):783-791.

Unit Design to Promote Healing

Physical Design for Safety

14. Bilchik GS. New vistas. Evidence-based design projects look into the links between a facility's environment and its care. *Health Facil Manage*. 2002;15(8):19-24.

15. Felver L. Patient-environment interactions in critical care. *Crit Care Nurs Clin N Am*. 1995;7(2):327-335.

16. Fontaine DK, Briggs LP, Pope-Smith B. Designing humanistic critical care environments. *Crit Care Nurs Q*. 2001;24(3):21-35.

17. Gallant D, Lanning K. Streamlining patient care processes through flexible room and equipment design. *Crit Care Nurs Q*. 2001;24(3):59-76.

18. Jastremski CA. ICU bedside environment. *Crit Care Clin*. 2000;16(4):723-735.

19. Long R. Healing by design. *Health Facil Manage*. 2001;11(4):20-22.

20. Lower J, Bonsack C. High-tech high touch: mission impossible? *Dimens Crit Care Nurs*. 2002;21(5):201-205.

21. Stichler JF. Creating healing environments in critical care units. *Crit Care Nurs Q*. 2001;24(3):1-21.

22. Williams M. Critical care unit design: a nursing perspective. *Crit Care Nurs Q*. 2001;24(3):35-43.

23. Bartley J, Bjerke NB. Infection control considerations in critical care unit design and construction: a systematic risk assessment. *Crit Care Nurs Q*. 2001;24(3):43-58.

24. Sehulster L, Chinn RY. Guidelines for environmental infection control in health-care facilities. Recommendations of CDC and Healthcare Infection Control Practices Advisory Committee. *MMWR*. 2003;52(RR-10):1-42.

Design for Psychological Well-Being

25. Cabrera IN, Lee MHM. Reducing noise pollution in the hospital setting by establishing a department of sound: a survey of recent research on the effects of noise and music in health care. *Prev Med*. 2000;30:339-345.

26. Cmiel CA, Karr DM, Gasser DM, et al. Noise control: a nursing team's approach to sleep promotion. *AJN*. 2004;104(2):40-48.

27. Edwards GB, Schuring L. Sleep protocol: a research-based practice change. *Crit Care Nurse*. 1993;13(2):84-88.

28. Evans D. The effectiveness of music as an intervention for hospital patients: a systematic review. *J Adv Nurs*. 2002;37(1):8-18.

29. Honkus VL. Sleep deprivation in critical care units. *Crit Care Nurs Q*. 2003;26(3):179-189.

30. NIH Technology Assessment Panel. Integration of behavioral and relaxation approaches into the treatment of chronic pain and insomnia. *JAMA*. 1996;276:313:318.

Healing Properties of Color and Light

31. Liberman J. *Light Medicine of the Future*. Rochester, Vt: Bear and Company Publishing; 1991.

32. Young-Mason J. The art of healing and healing power of art. *Clin Nurs Spec*. 14(4):196-197.

CLINICAL RECOMMENDATIONS

The rating scale for the Level of Recommendation ranges from I to VI, with levels indicated as follows: I, manufacturer's recommendations only; II, theory based, no research data to support recommendations; recommendations from expert consensus group may exist; III, laboratory data only, no clinical data to support recommendations; IV, limited clinical studies to support recommendations; V, clinical studies in more than 1 or 2 different populations and situations to support recommendations; VI, clinical studies in a variety of patient populations and situations to support recommendations.

Sphere of Influence	Recommendations	Rationale for Recommendation	Level of Recommendation	Supporting References	Comments
Organizational Culture for Healing	*Assessment*				
	Determine organizational commitment for developing an environment of healing using a systematic analysis of answers to crucial questions.	Whether you make a facility-based change or unit-based change, the answers to these questions will illuminate the challenges to be faced to be successful in instituting environmental changes that promote healing.	IV: Limited clinical studies to support recommendations	Annotated Bib: 1, 2 Suggested Readings: 6 Other References: 3-6	See Table 2 under General Description Section
	Interventions				
	Develop a committee to establish a written philosophy related to healing environments and to guide the introduction of specific projects related to healing environments.	This committee will determine the impact of proposed projects on all aspects of the organization.	II: Theory based, no research data to support recommendations; recommendations from expert consensus group may exist	Other References: 4, 6, 13, 14	
	Develop specific measures to evaluate the effect of healing environment projects. Measures of effectiveness should include clinical outcomes, financial effects, and patient/staff satisfaction.	Hospital administrators must be accountable for the expenditure of scarce resources. Measurements of effectiveness are important to demonstrate fiduciary responsibility and demonstrate designing for patient safety.	IV: Limited clinical studies to support recommendations	Annotated Bib: 2, 3, 5 Suggested Readings: 9, 11, 13, 15 Other References: 1-3, 8, 10, 11, 13, 21, 23	
	Consider participating in program projects that promote excellence in nursing such as the Magnet Program from the American Nurses Credentialing Center or adopting the AACN Synergy Model as a foundation for the provision of nursing and patient safety.	Programs like these require a thorough assessment of the organization's resources and commitment to excellence in patient care. This type of commitment reflects patient/family-centered care and innovation.	II: Theory based, no research data to support recommendations; recommendations from expert consensus group may exist	Annotated Bib: 4 Other References: 13	

Sphere of Influence	Recommendations	Rationale for Recommendation	Level of Recommendation	Supporting References	Comments
Unit/Area Design	*General Design* Gather specific guidelines to assist in making design plans. Guidelines include: SCCM Guidelines For Intensive Care Unit Design; Joint Commission on Accreditation of Healthcare Organizations' (JCAHO) Environment of Care Standards; CDC/HICPAC Guidelines for Environmental Control in Health-Care Facilities. Network and explore other facilities initiating similar projects such as those participating in the Pebble Project. Incorporate the following considerations important to healing designs that reduce stress: 1. Consider patients' social support. Design space for family and friends to provide support. Ensure comfortable furniture is available for family members. 2. Foster a sense of control in the design. Patients should be able to regulate their room temperature; when they have visitors; privacy (single rooms should be provided whenever possible); access to phone; access to distractions such as music, television, relaxing outside views; and easy to use bed and room controls. 3. Choose colors and artwork wisely. 4. Control acoustics to reduce the impact of hospital noise.	Evidence-based designs are proving to be not only safer, but more economical in terms of reducing risk and helping patients to heal faster and leave the hospital sooner.	IV: Limited clinical studies to support recommendations	Annotated Bib: 1-5 Suggested Readings: 13, 18, 20, 21, 23 Other References: 7, 15, 16, 19, 20, 22, 23	

Sphere of Influence	Recommendations	Rationale for Recommendation	Level of Recommendation	Supporting References	Comments
Unit/Area Design (***cont.***)	*General Design (cont.)*				
	5. Consider designs that streamline patient care processes and reduce moving patients from area to area (acuity-adaptable room designs).				
	Consider holding design meetings in a mock patient room.	Helps clinicians and nonclinicians visualize issues of importance			
	Design for Safety				
	Critical care units with the following design elements reduce exposure to infection and injury, reduce patient transfers and resultant medical errors and increased lengths of stay, and increase patient and staff satisfaction:	Acuity-based room designs reduce the labor costs and potential for medical errors of patient transfers. Private rooms decrease exposure to hospital-acquired infections and promote better sleep and better family support. Full-spectrum lighting enhances well-being. A centralized nurses' station allows for better visibility to reduce patient injury and facilitate early intervention for problems. Patient control of temperature and lights allows for better sleep. Noise abatement features on equipment and policies to decrease noxious noise facilitate sleep and decrease exposure to harmful decibel levels. All factors increase staff and patient/family satisfaction and assist in maintaining the patients normal rhythmic patterns.	IV: Limited clinical studies to support recommendations	Annotated Bib: 7, 9, 10 Suggested Readings: 13, 20, 21 Other references: 7, 16, 40, 61, 64	
	• Private rooms with space to accommodate families				
	• Centralized nurses station				
	• Acuity-adaptive room designs				
	• Patient control of temperature and light				
	• State-of-the-art beds that weigh patients and equipment that minimizes noxious noise.				
	• Full-spectrum lighting should be available as well as natural lighting from windows. Lighting in the room should be able to be controlled by the patient. In addition, there should be lighting designed for procedures and nighttime lighting for safety and monitoring.				
	• Noise abatement equipment and policies				

Sphere of Influence	Recommendations	Rationale for Recommendation	Level of Recommendation	Supporting References	Comments
Unit/Area Design *(cont.)*	*Infection Control* There is limited evidence that specific design issues have a direct outcome on nosocomial infections. However, private rooms, good air quality maintenance, and effective hand washing do limit the patient's risks. Therefore the following considerations should be given to unit design and hospital policy related to infection control: • Private rooms should be used whenever possible and must be used appropriately for isolation cases. • Consider acuity-adaptable rooms to decrease patient movement throughout the hospitalization. • Provide alcohol-based hand sanitizers in areas not easily accessible to sinks. • Post signs encouraging patients/families to remind staff to wash their hands before touching the patient. • Ensure hand washing facilities are readily accessible to patient rooms. • Consider developing programs to sensitize staff to proper cleaning of personal equipment such as stethoscopes, pagers, cell phones, etc. • Develop policies to limit using such personal equipment in patient rooms, particularly in rooms of highly compromised patients.	Antibiotic-resistant infections are life threatening to the vulnerable critical care population.	IV: Limited clinical studies to support recommendations	Annotated Bib: 6 Suggested Readings: 13, 22, 23, 30 Other references: 24-28	

Sphere of Influence	Recommendations	Rationale for Recommendation	Level of Recommendation	Supporting References	Comments
Unit/Area Design *(cont.)*	*Infection Control* *(cont.)* • Use cohort staffing (patient care staff use is limited to one or two staff members a shift; all others who provide care must change clothes prior to caring for other patients) to limit the spread of highly contagious, antibiotic-resistant infections such as MRSA, *Aspergillus*, and *Acinetobacter*. *Noise Abatement Protocol* • Conduct an assessment of noise levels at various times in the unit using a decibel meter. • Based on this assessment, plan for interventions to decrease noise such as: 　• Closing doors to patient rooms. 　• On-going staff education program to sensitize staff to the level of noise created by conversations and routine practices. 　• Using bedside small televisions and pillow speakers rather than wall-mounted larger televisions. 　• Evaluating alarms systems when purchasing equipment. 　• Decreasing the volume of telephone ringers. 　• Limiting overhead paging or paging in all rooms over the call system to emergencies only. 　• Ensuring administrative processes such as using addressographs and opening and closing chart binders are	High noise levels are detrimental to patients; healing can be delayed, anxiety increased, and sleep disrupted. There is a potential for hearing loss with prolonged exposure to high decibels during care. Developing a specific unit plan to address noise abatement is best accomplished when unit data collected indicates the need. Some noise cannot be eliminated such as factory set alarms designed to alert staff to emergencies. However, behavior can be modified to reduce the level of noise in critical care units.	V: Clinical studies in more than 1 or 2 different populations and situations to support recommendations	Annotated Bib: 9, 10 Suggested Readings: 24, 25 Other References: 29, 40, 43, 44, 47, 52-55	

Sphere of Influence	Recommendations	Rationale for Recommendation	Level of Recommendation	Supporting References	Comments
Unit/Area Design *(cont.)*	*Noise Abatement Protocol (cont.)* minimized during nighttime. • Considering purchasing electric versus manual addressographs. • Monitoring family visiting with patient and coordinating family presence and education to ensure periods of rest free from conversation. • Considering the use of earplugs and/or music therapy to decrease the effects of noxious sound stimuli.				
Design for Psychological Well-Being	*Music Therapy to Promote Rest and Relaxation* • When using music to reduce anxiety and promote rest and relaxation, allow patients to control the type of music and duration of listening. If patients cannot do this, obtain input from family. • Avoid the use of live music in the unit—it may disrupt or contribute to the stress of others. • Do not using music for prolonged periods; usually periods of 1-2 hrs duration is sufficient. • Ensure that music is provided through a mechanism such as head phones or in private rooms where it will not disturb others.	Evidence exists that music therapy promotes relaxation, decreases anxiety, and promotes sleep. There is not good evidence that it decreases pain due to painful procedures. Music therapy works best in measured doses and when it is patient controlled.	VI: Clinical studies in a variety of patient populations and situations to support recommendations	Annotated Bib: 11-14 Suggested Readings: 15, 17, 22, 27 Other References: 30-39, 41, 45-48, 50, 51, 56-58	

Sphere of Influence	Recommendations	Rationale for Recommendation	Level of Recommendation	Supporting References	Comments
Design for Psychological Well-Being *(cont.)*	*Healing Properties of Color, Light, and Art* • Whenever possible, provide the patient with an aesthetic view from a window that provides natural daylight and exposure to light-dark cycles. • Consider placement of gardens on hospital grounds so that they are viewed from patient rooms. • Choose appropriate colors for patient rooms. Red, orange, and yellow tend to increase blood pressure and heart and respiratory rates, while green, blue, and black decrease them. Using moderate warm colors without sharp contrasts to promote rest. • Color can be introduced through the use of art on the walls of patient rooms. Evidence suggests that pastoral and water scenes are most soothing. Avoid the use of abstract art with bold colors and rectilinear forms. • Using a committee to select or accept art from donations may assist in ensuring art that reduces anxiety and promotes a feeling of well-being. Typically, certain themes should be avoided in patient rooms, such as portraits and religious themes.	Color, light, and art are ancient forms of healing. There is evidence that patients heal faster when they have access to natural light or full-spectrum light and there is appropriate art work in patient rooms. Gardens are an excellent way to bring color, light, and art to patients through a room with a view.	IV: Limited clinical studies to support recommendations	Annotated Bib: 21, 22 Suggested Readings: 15, 30, 31 Other References: 59-66	

Sphere of Influence	Recommendations	Rationale for Recommendation	Level of Recommendation	Supporting References	Comments
Acute and Critical Care Patients	*Protocol to Promote Sleep with Nonpharmacologic interventions*				
	• Ensure that unit staff are adequately educated about the negative effects of sleep deprivation and the positive effects of a protocol to promote sleep.	Evidence indicates that pharmacologic methods of promoting sleep can be reduced with nonpharmacologic interventions. It is important to ensure that acute and critically ill patients are appropriately medicated for pain, anxiety, or symptoms of delirium. However, nonpharmacologic methods can reduce the need for medication or decrease the dose of medication needed.	V: Clinical studies in more than 1 or 2 different populations and situations to support recommendations	Annotated Bib: 7, 10, 14-20 Suggested Readings 25, 26, 28 Other References: 49, 50, 51, 53, 55	
	• Assess patient for individual risks for sleep disturbance: pain, anxiety, history of impaired sleep, inability to perform usual nighttime regimen.				
	• Initiate unit processes to reduce noise.				
	• Offer patient option of brushing teeth, washing face, and/or having a back rub.	A consistent plan to promote sleep is essential to ensure that adequate cycles of REM sleep occur and that the patient does not suffer the consequences of fatigue and stress that occur without adequate periods of rest.			
	• Provide measures to reduce pain and anxiety such as message therapy or guided imagery.				
	• Prepare patient room for sleep: reduce lighting, offer music intervention or sound therapy; offer ear plugs or sleep masks if appropriate; close door to room; post sign that patient is resting.				
	• Decrease interruptions to sleep; block out times for no interruptions for medications or tests if possible.				

ANNOTATED BIBLIOGRAPHY

Organizational Culture for Healing

1. Gerteis M, Edgman-Levitan S, Daley J, Delbanco TL. *Through the Patient's Eyes. Understanding and Promoting Patient-Centered Care.* San Francisco, Calif: Jossey-Bass; 1993.

Study Sample

Survey data obtained from 6000 patients and 2000 family members obtained during 62 hospital visits to 20 different hospitals.

Comparison Studied

A descriptive study evaluating the experiences of hospitalized patients and families. Methodologies included extensive literature review, focus group interviews, and written survey analysis.

Study Procedures

This study was funded by the Picker/Commonwealth Program for Patient-Centered Care through the Commonwealth Fund of New York. The goal was to explore the patients' needs as they defined them based on being hospitalized. Focus groups and literature review revealed 7 dimensions of patient-centered care: (1) respect for patient's values, preferences, and expressed needs; (2) coordination and integration of care; (3) information, communication, and education; (4) physical comfort; (5) emotional support and alleviation of fear and anxiety; (6) involvement of family and friends; and (7) transition and continuity. Program consultants, using a survey instrument designed to elicit reports from patients and their care partners, interviewed 6000 patients recently hospitalized and 2000 care partners randomly selected from 62 hospitals nationwide. Consultants also visited more than 20 hospitals, including exemplary ones and those that scored high or low on the survey.

Key Results

Each chapter in the book integrates the results of the literature review and survey finding related to each of the 7 dimensions. Conclusions included:

1. The quality of patient-centered hospital care is an institutional characteristic that transcends any particular program or activity.
2. Some environments are more conducive to patient-centered care than others. Almost all the top performing hospitals were not teaching hospitals.
3. Management is critical to performance, regardless of the environment.

Study Strengths and Weaknesses

National study with random selection of patients across numerous hospitals. Extensive review of the literature integrated into analysis of prospective qualitative and quantitative data obtained with a variety of methodologies. A classic study.

Clinical Implications

All health care providers should read the results of this study. Until we understand what is important to patients, designing systems of healing with an organizational culture of healing cannot succeed.

2. Malloch K. Healing models for organizations: description, measurement, and outcomes. *J Healthcare Manag.* 2000;45(5):332-345.

Study Sample

This study evaluated 3 elements of a healing model for organizations in the context of one 100-bed facility known for its healing environment. One hundred ninety-two employees participated; 76 RNs and 116 nonregistered nurses.

Comparison Studied

The overall purpose was to explore the relationships between overall job satisfaction and staff perceptions of the extent to which the healing model incorporates common understanding of health as a mind-body-spirit interrelationship, patient-centered relationships, and a culture supportive of personal growth and mastery. Trends of organizational performance were compared to regional norms.

Four hypotheses were examined:

1. The greater the staff perceptions of a wellness orientation, the greater their job satisfaction.
2. The greater the staff perceptions of the presence of caring relationships, the greater their job satisfaction.
3. The greater the staff perceptions of the presence of an organizational culture supportive of personal growth and mastery, the greater their job satisfaction.
4. The combination of these 3 healing model variables will explain a greater proportion of variation in job satisfaction than any single variable.

Study Procedures

A descriptive correlational survey design was used to evaluate the 4 study hypotheses. Case study time-series analysis methods were used to examine the secondary aims of comparing trends to regional norms. Four standard survey instruments were used and one Healing Context Demographic Information Questionnaire was developed for the study.

Key Results

Significant correlations supported all 4 hypotheses. Of the responding employees, 72% (136) had an orientation to wellness. Seven healing variables (in order: supervisor support, clarity of expectations, involvement of employees, peer cohesion, innovation, health conceptions, and caring) were statistically correlated to job satisfaction (r = .27 to .57, $P < .001$). Regression analysis indicated synergistic effects explaining 45% of the variance in job satisfaction was due to 4 variables (supervisor support, involvement of employees, wellness orientation, and clarity of expectations).

Study Strengths and Weaknesses

This is one of the first studies of a healing model using measures of healing environment variables. Findings can only be generalized to the single location of the study.

Clinical Implications

Healing environments are important to patients and families and are cost-effective for organizations. Developing an organizational model for creating a healing environment will assist in designing and evaluating such environments. More research is needed in this area.

3. **Martin DP, Diehr P, Conrad DA, Davis JH, Keickly R, Perrin EB. Randomized trial of a patient-centered hospital unit.** *Patient and Educ Counsel.* **1998;34:125-133.**

Study Sample

Seven hundred sixty patients randomized into a Planetree model medical-surgical unit for care (n = 315) or one of 4 other traditional medical-surgical units for care (n = 445) in one hospital in San Francisco, Calif.

Comparison Studied

The hypothesis was that a stay in the Planetree unit would improve outcomes of care related to patient satisfaction, health education, patient involvement in care, health behaviors, perceived health status, and use of services.

Study Procedures

Patients 18 years of age or older who understood English and were well enough to complete an admission interview were randomized into the Planetree group or traditional group. They were randomized in blocks of 20; however, there was cross-assignment into units due to the high occupancy rate. Because there were no statistically significant differences in demographic information between randomized and nonrandomized patients into any of the units, the two groups of patients were combined for each arm of the study (ie, Planetree and traditional group). Study patients (85% of those eligible) were significantly younger than those who declined to participate. Each patient completed a 20-minute interview at admission, a questionnaire 1 week after discharge to assess short-term effects of hospitalization, and questionnaires at 3 and 6 months postdischarge to assess any longer-term affects on outcomes. Chi square or *t* test analysis was used to compare patient characteristics.

Outcome variables were analyzed with analysis of covariance. Adjustments were made for case mix and severity.

Key Results

Planetree participants were significantly older, had a lower level of education, and worked fewer hours full-time. All other patient characteristics were nonsignificant between the groups. Although Planetree units had significantly more health education during the stay, health behavior outcomes were not statistically different between the groups, nor were differences in patient control over health or coping strategies. Hospital resource utilization also did not vary significantly. Planetree patients were significantly more satisfied with their stay and with patient education.

Study Strengths and Weaknesses

A strength is the prospective, randomized design of the trial. Health status measurements were evaluated using reliable and valid scales. Scales used for assessing coping and control over health were not well described but were described as having lower reliability and validity than other measures. Only 1 facility was used, thus limiting generalization of results.

Clinical Implications

The authors acknowledge that hospital stays may be too short to provide time for patients to absorb needed education and strategies for making changes to lifelong habits and behaviors. Continuity of education is likely needed to promote long-term health behavior changes. Planetree units appear to not require greater resources, and patient satisfaction was higher in Planetree units. More research should be done involving other aspects of this healing environment in acute care.

4. **Muenzen PM, Greenberg S.** *Results of the AACN Certification Corporation Study of Practice.* **New York, NY: Professional Examination Service; 1997.**

Study Sample

Surveys sent to 3924 nurses (adult, pediatric, and neonatal nurses in subacute, acute, and critical care settings) with a 24% response rate.

Comparison Studied

Descriptive survey research to delineate the validity of the AACN Synergy Model as a valid descriptor of acute and critical care practice.

Study Procedures

Surveys asked participants to read patient care scenarios and rank the level of patient function (on a scale of 1 = lowest level of function to 5 = highest level of function) based on 8 distinct characteristics described in the Synergy Model.

Then, based on the patient's needs as described by the level of function on the 8 characteristics, determine the level of competency of the nurse for 8 characteristics of practice based on a similar rating scale.

Key Results

- Respondents accurately perceived patient acuity in the profiles developed for the study.
- Respondents perceived that patients with more acute care need profiles required higher levels of nurse characteristics of practice than profiles of less acutely ill patients.
- Clinical judgment was the nurse characteristic that was most strongly related to patient need.
- The 8 patient characteristics and their associated rating scales were useful in differentiating patient acuity levels.
- Acuity of care levels were not differentiated based on the patient/family's ability to participate in decision making and care nor were they differentiated by the patient/family's level of technical, fiscal, personal, and psychological/social resources.
- Critical care patients are not found solely in critical care units.
- The 8 patient characteristics fall into 2 groups: intrinsic and extrinsic.
- The 8 nurse characteristics are all intercorrelated and may reflect overall nurse competency.

Study Strengths and Weaknesses

Although response rate was low, the volume of responses was adequate for appropriate statistical analysis. This is a strong, statistically valid analysis of a humane, caring model of nursing practice that matches nurse competencies to specific needs of patients/families.

Clinical Implications

Although the Synergy Model is a valid model to describe actual practice, more research is needed to measure patient and organizational outcomes when using the model.

5. Rubin HR, Owens AJ, Golden G. *Status Report (1998): An Investigation to Determine Whether the Built Environment Affects Patients' Medical Outcomes*. Martinez, Calif: The Center for Health Design Inc; 1998.

Study Sample

Eighty-four published studies that indicate a measurable relationship between the environment of care and patient outcomes.

Comparison Studied

This report reflects work contracted by the Center for Health Design and done by the Quality of Care Research department at Johns Hopkins University. The project began in 1995, and

work was updated in 1998. Originally, there were 3 tasks: (1) review the literature to find out what is known about the effect of the health care environmental design on patient health outcomes; (2) suggest design application based on the literature review; and (3) make initial recommendation for developing a research agenda in this area for the next 10 or more years. The work was updated in 1998 to expand the literature review and conduct focus groups to help choose subjects for the study of effects of environment on medical outcomes.

Study Procedures

Literature review and analysis, focus group interviews.

Key Results

Seventy-four of the studies (88%) indicated that some environmental feature was related to patient outcomes. However, 39 of them had a weak design. Forty-five studies (82%) of studies with a stronger design also found positive correlations. There was no statistical difference between the proportion of strong to weak studies ($P > .075$). Three conclusions were made based on the analysis of the body of existing research: 1) based on the few strong studies reviewed, improvements in outcomes may be available through design interventions guided by sound scientific inquiry; 2) studies that contain data about the effect of the environment on health outcomes are scarce; and 3) many published studies have significant methodological flaws that render their conclusions suspect or cast doubt on the generalizability of their findings.

Study Strengths and Weaknesses

A comprehensive review of the literature searching for outcomes related to environmental factors. Search strategy was well conceived, and studies were analyzed with stringent criteria. An annotated bibliography of studies is provided including the strengths and weaknesses of the studies. A future research agenda is provided.

Clinical Implications

The difficulty of designing studies to measure outcomes of environmental design is highlighted by this review. However, with advances in research design, better studies are possible and need to be conducted. We have an ethical obligation to not harm patients, and it is becoming clear that hospital design and organizational culture can harm patients. It is also becoming more evident that healing environments do affect outcomes positively.

Environmental Design for Healing

6. Dettenkofer M, Seegers MD, Antes G, et al. Does the architecture of hospital facilities influence nosocomial infection rates? A systematic review. *Infect Control Hosp Epidemiol.* 2004;25(1):21-25.

Study Sample

Review of 178 published studies dated from 1975-2001.

Comparison Studied

To review scientific literature for evidence of the effects of interventions to improve hospital design and construction on the occurrence of nosocomial infections.

Study Procedures

Medline, Science Citation Index/Web of Science, Current Contents, Heclinet, Healthstar, Somed, and Embase databases were searched for the years 1975-2001 using the following keywords or combinations: (build*, rebuild*, renov*, construct*, or architect*) and hospital*; and (infect*, hygien*, bacter*, contamin*, or transmiss*). Bibliographies of all reviewed papers were searched by hand and experts were contacted. Criteria were used for assessing the strength of evidence ranging from I = Meta-analysis based on randomized, controlled trials to V = Expert judgment, consensus statements, and reports. Data were validated by using 2 independent reviewers to screen all abstracts and 2 reviewers to critically appraise the studies and reports. Reports graded as IV or V were not considered in the final assessment of evidence. If reviewers disagreed, a third reviewer's perspective was obtained and a joint opinion by all 3 was reached.

Key Results

Three hundred eighty-two articles were retrieved, and 178 meeting the inclusion criteria were identified and evaluated (ICU = 41; surgical departments = 83; isolation units = 7; hospitals in general = 47). Only 17 of the 178 described completed concurrent or historical cohort studies matching the criteria for final inclusion (ICU, 9; surgical departments, 4; isolation units, 2; hospitals in general, 2). None included a meta-analysis systematic review or randomized, controlled trial. Interventions usually included a move to new location or renovation. Also, there usually was an increase in staff-to-patient ratio along with the moves or renovation. Conclusion: the lack of evidence is related to multifactoral nature of nosocomial infections. Some improvement will be seen with increased space, isolation capacity, and improved hand-washing facilities. Improper hand washing may have a greater impact on nosocomial infections than the architecture of the facility.

Study Strengths and Weaknesses

Outstanding example of a systematic review of literature to determine evidence-based practice.

Clinical Implications

Many interventions should be used to prevent nosocomial infections. Hand washing is the simplest and most economical. However, more systematic, well-controlled studies should be designed to look at the impact of architecture physical factors and on staff practices that lead to nosocomial infections.

Design for Psychological Well-Being

7. **Kahn DM, Cook TE, Carlisle CC, et al. Identification and modification of environmental noise in an ICU setting. *Chest*. 1998;114(2):535-540.**

Study Sample

All ICU staff during the study period in the medical intensive care or respiratory intensive care units of a 720-bed teaching hospital in Providence, RI.

Comparison Studied

Phase I identified what individual noises were causing the high peak sound levels observed in previous studies. Phase II reduced the number of sound peaks greater than 80 dBA in the MICU through the implementation of a noise behavior modification program with ICU staff.

Study Procedures

In phase I measurements were made on 16 separate occasions. Peak sound levels were measured for 15-second intervals for 10 consecutive minutes. A single observer sat at the head of the bed and used a calibrated sound lever meter to simultaneously record sound peaks while subjectively identifying the source of the loudest noise heard. Prior to making the observations, the observer had a hearing test indicating normal frequency hearing.

In phase II, baseline noise levels were measured over several days in the MICU using 60-second intervals. Both in phase I and phase II the time blocks for measurement were 6 AM-12 PM and 12 AM to 6 AM. A single 3-bed room was used and data were collected about the patients' severity of illness and number of devices in use during the baseline measurements. Once baseline data were collected, an educational behavior modification program was initiated with all the staff, to include physicians, nurses, therapists, and secretaries. Topics included information about noise pollution and its impact on patients and on the work environment. The causes of noise pollution felt to be most amenable to behavior modification were television, talking, beepers, and the intercom system. The behavior modification education program lasted 3 weeks. Data were recorded on 2 baseline days and 2 days after receiving the behavior modification program.

Key Results

In phase I, 12 noises were identified as contributing to high peak sound levels. Fifty-one percent were potentially modifiable, television and talking being the dominant causes. In phase 2, the mean peak sound levels were very high before and at the end of the trial of behavior modification (80.0 ± 0.1 dBA and 78.1 ± 0.1 dBA respectively). The change was significant at the $P = .0001$ level. The noise levels actually increased during the 12 AM to 6 AM time period.

Study Strengths and Weaknesses

Attempts were made to control the many variables that effect the measurements in this study. The length of time of measurement postbehavior modification was not reported. Although the modification program statistically decreased noise levels, they still remained above EPA recommended levels.

Clinical Implications

This study reinforced the various types of ICU noises that exceed recommended levels. Behavior modification strategies used did decrease noise but not to levels that reflect EPA guidelines. However, many useful strategies to reduce noise were used. Noise levels at night remain very problematic.

8. Chlan L, Tracy MF, Nelson B, et al. Feasibility of a music intervention protocol for patients receiving mechanical ventilatory support. *Altern Ther Health Med.* 2001;7(6):80-83.

Study Sample

Five alert critically ill adults receiving mechanical ventilatory support.

Comparison Studied

Descriptive pilot study to test the feasibility of a patient-initiated music intervention protocol.

Study Procedures

Study conducted in 2 adult critical care units in a university-affiliated tertiary care center in the urban Midwest. Patients listened to audiotaped music they selected through head phones over a period of 3 days. The patients determined the length of each session and the frequency of sessions. Heart rate, respiratory rate, blood pressure, anxiety, and identified barriers to protocol adherence were outcomes measured.

Key Results

Patients averaged 2 self-initiated sessions lasting approximately 68 minutes per session. Barriers included inaccessibility of the equipment and lack of knowledge and experience of the staff. Physiological variables were not analyzed due to missing data.

Study Strengths and Weaknesses

Pilot design to determine parameters for designing a more comprehensive comparative study. Good description of barriers and problems in measuring outcomes.

Clinical Implications

Allowing patients choices to control their environment continues to reduce anxiety. Music interventions controlled by patients can assist in reducing anxiety and promoting relaxation.

9. Tamburri LM, DiBrienza R, Zozula R, et al. Nocturnal care interactions with patients in critical care units. *Am J Crit Care.* 2004;13(2): 102-115.

Study Sample

Medical records of 50 patients age 21 or older admitted to 4 critical care units of a university-affiliated tertiary care medical center in the northeastern United States. The 4 units were a 16-bed MICU, 8-bed CCU, 7-bed neurosurgical ICU, and 10-bed surgical/trauma ICU. Records of patients who were undergoing treatment with neuromuscular blocking agents, intra-aortic balloon pumps, or continuous venovenous hemofiltration were not included due to the continuous bedside care requirements.

Comparison Studied

The following questions were addressed:

1. What are the frequency, patterns, and types of nocturnal care interactions with critically ill patients?
2. What are the relationships between patients' acuity, age, sex, and the frequency of nocturnal care interactions among critically ill patients?
3. What are the differences in the frequency of, patterns of, and types of nocturnal care interactions between patients admitted to ICUs being studied?

Data were collected for the time frame of 7 PM to 7 AM using a checklist developed by the researchers.

Study Procedures

Data about care activities were collected by 2 clinical nurse specialists using an investigator checklist. Open medical records of patients who stayed in the ICU for 4 consecutive nights were reviewed on randomly chosen days. The first night the patient stayed in the unit was not included.

Key Results

Data consisted of interactions during 147 nights. The mean number of care interactions per night was 42.6, with interactions most frequent at midnight and less at 3 AM. Only 9 periods of uninterrupted periods of sleep (2-3 hours) were available (6% of the 147 nights studied). Frequency of interactions correlated significantly with patient acuity. One sleep promotion intervention was documented in the 147 nights, and 62% of routine daily baths were provided between 9 PM and 6 AM. Sixty-one percent of these occurred between 2 AM and 5 AM.

Study Strengths and Weaknesses

Good preparation to develop a sleep promotion protocol for prospective study. Retrospective design limited the quality and availability of data collected. Sleep was not measured.

Clinical Implications

This study emphasizes the continued pattern of routine care practices despite evidence that such practice may delay healing. Giving baths and interrupting sleep for standard monitoring protocols needs to be examined in light of the individual patient's needs.

10. Ulrich RS, Lundén O, Eltinge JL. Effects of exposure to nature and abstract pictures on patients recovering from open heart surgery. *Psychophysiology*. 1993;37:S7.

Study Sample

One hundred and sixty-six patients who underwent an open-heart surgery in a Swedish hospital.

Comparison Studied

Comparison of response to visual stimulation by a nature picture dominated by either water or trees, and abstract picture dominated by either curvilinear or rectilinear forms, or a control condition consisting of either a white pane or no picture at all.

Study Procedures

Participants were randomly assigned to 1 of 6 groups with either one of the nature, abstract, or control pictures placed at the foot of the bed in the ICU postsurgery. Variables were collected presurgery, during the ICU stay, and through the ward phase until discharge.

Key Results

Self-ratings indicated patients exposed to an open view of water experienced less postoperative anxiety than patients in any of the other 5 groups ($P < .01$). These patients required fewer doses of strong pain medications during the ward phase, but received more frequent doses of moderate strength pain medication. Across all picture categories, negative ratings were associated with increased intake of strong pain medication. Several patients had strong reactions to the rectilinear abstract art, requiring its removal.

Study Strengths and Weaknesses

Only an abstract of this study is published making it impossible to replicate study procedures not well described. Strong design and sample size.

Clinical Implications

Natural environment pictures may contribute to positive outcomes of recovery from open-heart surgery. Art committees need to be cautious in using abstract art in patient rooms.

OTHER REFERENCES

Organizational Culture of Healing

1. Baggs JG, Ryan SA, Phelps CE, et al. The association between interdisciplinary collaboration and patient outcomes in a medical intensive care unit. *Heart Lung*. 1992;21:18-24.
2. Carson SS, Stocking C, Podsadecki T, et al. Effects of organizational change in the medical intensive care unit of a teaching hospital. *JAMA*. 1996;276(4):322-328.
3. Fottler MD, Ford RC, Roberts V, et al. Creating a healing environment: the importance of the service setting in the new consumer-oriented healthcare system. *J Health Manag*. 2000;45(2):91-106.
4. Geary H. Facilitating an organizational culture of healing in an urban medical center. *Nurs Admin Q*. 2003; 27(3):231-239.
5. Goe SJ. Beyond waterfalls and grand pianos. *Health Exec*. 2003;18(4):68-69.
6. Huelat BJ. 10 myths of healing environments. *Health Facil Manag*. 1998;11(2):24-30.
7. Jastremski CA. Making changes to improve the intensive care unit experience for patients and their families. *New Horiz*. 1998;6(1):99-109.
8. Knaus WA, Draper EA, Wagner DP, et al. An evaluation of outcome from intensive care in major medical centers. *Ann Intern Med*. 1986;104:410-418.
9. Kritek PB. Rethinking the critical care environment: luxury or necessity? *AACN Clin Issues*. 2001;12(3): 336-344.
10. Mitchell PH, Armstrong S, Simpson TF, et al. American Association of Critical-Care Nurses Demonstration Project: profile of excellence in critical care nursing. *Heart Lung*. 1989;18:19-27.
11. Mitchell PH, Shannon SE, Cain KC, et al. Critical care outcomes: linking structures, processes, and organizational and clinical outcomes. *Am J Crit Care*. 1996;5: 353-363.
12. Pettigrew J. Intensive care nursing. The ministry of presence. *Crit Care Nurs Clin N Am*. 1990;2(3):503-508.
13. Robinson CA. Magnet nursing services recognition: transforming the critical care environment. *AACN Clin Issues*. 2001;12(3):411-423.
14. Romano M. Slow growing. Planetree philosophy sprouts new branches of support but remains on the healthcare periphery. *Mod Health*. 2002;32(32):30-33.

Environment Design for Healing

15. American College of Medicine/Society of Critical Care Medicine. Guidelines for intensive care unit design. *Crit Care Med*. 1995;23(3):582-588.
16. American Institute of Architects. *2001 Guidelines for Design and Construction of Hospitals and Healthcare Facilities*. Washington DC: The American Institute of Architects Press; 2001.

17. Burmahl B. Future is now. *Health Facil Manage.* 2002;15(3):16-22.

18. Joint Commission on Accreditation of Healthcare Organizations. *2005 Comprehensive Accreditation Manual for Hospitals: The Official Handbook.* Oakbrook Terrace, Ill: JCAHO; 2005.

19. Murphy E. The patient room of the future. *Nurs Manage.* 2000;31(3):38-39.

20. Pangrazio JR. Room with a view. Looking at the future of patient room design. *Health Facil Manage.* 2003;16(12):30-32.

21. Runy LA. Best practices and safety issues in the ICU. *Hosp Health Net.* 2004;78(4):45-51.

22. Ulrich RS. How design impacts wellness. *Health Forum J.* 1992;35:20-25.

23. Voelker R. "Pebbles" cast ripples in health care design. *JAMA.* 2001;286(14):1701-1702.

24. Bayat A, Shaaban H, Dodgson A, et al. Implications for burns unit design following outbreak of multi-resistant *Acinetobacter* infection in ICU and burns unit. *Burns.* 2003;29:303-306.

25. Carducci A, Verani M, Casini B, et al. Detection and potential indicators of the presence of hepatitis C virus on surfaces in hospital settings. *Letters Appl Microbio.* 2002;34(3):189-193.

26. Cotterill S, Evans R, Fraise AP. An unusual source for an outbreak of methicillin-resistant *Staphylococcus aureus* on an intensive therapy unit. *J Hosp Infect.* 1996;32:207-216.

27. Humphreys H, Johnson EM, Warnock DW, et al. An outbreak of aspergillosis in a general ITU. *J Hosp Infect.* 1991;18:167-177.

28. Noskin GA, Peterson LR. Engineering infection control through facility design. *Emerging Infectious Dis.* 2001;7(2):354-357.

Design for Psychological Well-Being

29. Aaron JN, Carlisle CC, Carskadon MA, et al. Environmental noise as a cause of sleep disruption in an intermediate care unit. *Sleep.* 1996;19:707-710.

30. Allaouchiche B, Duflo F, Debon R, et al. Noise in the postanesthesia care unit. *Brit J Anesth.* 2002;88(3):369-373.

31. Baker CF, Garvin BJ, Kennedy CW, et al. The effect of environmental sound and communication on CCU patients' heart rate and blood pressure. *Res Nurs & Health.* 1993;16:415-421.

32. Bally K, Campbell D, Chesnick K, et al. Effects of patient-controlled music therapy during coronary angiography on procedural pain and anxiety distress syndrome. *Crit Care Nurse.* 2003;23(2):50-58.

33. Barnason S, Zimmerman L, Nieveen J. The effects of music interventions on anxiety in the patient after coronary artery bypass grafting. *Heart Lung.* 1995;24:124-132.

34. Bolwerk CA. Effects of relaxing music on state anxiety in myocardial infarction patients. *Crit Care Nurs Q.* 1990;13(2):66-73.

35. Cadigan ME, Caruso NA, Halderman SM, et al. The effects of music on cardiac patients on bed rest. *Prog Cardiovasc Nurse.* 2001;16(1):5-13.

36. Chlan L, Tracy MF. Music therapy in critical care: indications and guidelines for intervention. *Crit Care Nurse.* 1999;19(3):35-41.

37. Chlan LL. Music therapy as a nursing intervention for patients supported by mechanical ventilation. *AACN Clin Issues.* 2000;11(1):128-138.

38. Davis-Rollans D, Cunningham SG. Physiologic responses of coronary care patients to selected music. *Heart Lung.* 1987;16:370-378.

39. Dossey L. Taking note: music, mind, and nature. *Altern Ther Health Med.* 2003;9(4):10-4, 94-100.

40. Dreher HM. Beyond stages of sleep: an emerging nursing model of sleep phases. *Holist Nurs Pract.* 1996;10(4):1-11.

41. Ferguson SL, Voll KV. Burn pain and anxiety: the use of music relaxation during rehabilitation. *J Burn Care Rehabil.* 2004;25(1):8-14.

42. Fontaine D. Measurement of nocturnal sleep patterns in trauma patients. *Heart Lung.* 1989;18:402-410.

43. Gagner-Tjellesen D, Yurkovich EE, Gragert M. Use of music therapy and other ITNIs in acute care. *J Psychosoc Nurs Ment Health Serv.* 2001;39(10):26-37.

44. Guzzetta CE. Effects of relaxation and music therapy on patients in a coronary care unit with presumptive acute myocardial infarction. *Heart Lung.* 1989;18:609-616.

45. Hanser SB, Mandel SE. The effects of music therapy in cardiac healthcare. *Cardiol Rev.* 2005;13(1):18-23.

46. Hilton A. Noise in acute patient care areas. *Res Nurs Health.* 1985;8:283-291.

47. McCaffrey RG, Good M. The lived experience of listening to music while recovering from surgery. *J Holist Nurs.* 2000;18(4):378-390.

48. McCarthy DO, Ouimet ME, Daun JM. Shades of Florence Nightingale: Potential impact of noise stress on wound healing. *Holistic Nurs Pract.* 1991;5(4):39-48.

49. Meyer-Falcke A, Rack R, Eichwede F, et al. How noisy are anaesthesia and intensive care medicine? Quantification of the patients' stress. *Eur J Anaesth.* 1994;11:407-411.

50. Meyer TJ, Eveloff SE, Bauer MS, et al. Adverse environmental conditions in the respiratory and medical ICU settings. *Chest.* 1994;105:1211-1216.

51. Moore MM, Nguyen D, Nolan SP, et al. Interventions to reduce decibel levels on patient care units. *Am Surg.* 1998;64:894-899.

52. Nilsson U, Rawal N, Enqvist B, et al. Analgesia following music and therapeutic suggestions in the PACU in ambulatory surgery; a randomized controlled trial. *Acta Anaesthesiol Scand.* 2003;47(3):278-283.

53. Nilsson U, Rawal N, Unosson M. A comparison of intra-operative or postoperative exposure to music—a controlled trial of the effects on postoperative pain. *Anaesthesia.* 2003;58(7):699-703.

54. Olson DM, Borel CO, Laskowitz DT, et al. Quiet time: a nursing intervention to promote sleep in neurocritical care units. *Am J Crit Care.* 2001;10(2):74-78.

55. Pope DS. Music, noise, and the human voice in the nurse-patient environment. *Image: J Nurs Scholars.* 1995;27(4):291-296.

56. Prensner JD, Yowler CJ, Smith LF, et al. Music therapy for assistance with pain and anxiety management in burn treatment. *J Burn Care Rehab.* 2001;22(1):83-88.

57. Pulling CA. The relationship between critical care nurses' knowledge about sleep and the initiation of sleep-promoting interventions. *AXON.* 1991;13(2):57-62.

58. Reimer M. Sleep pattern disturbance: nursing interventions perceived by patients and their nurses as facilitating nocturnal sleep in the hospital. In: McLane A. (Ed.) *Classification of Nursing Diagnoses: Proceedings of the 7th Conference, St Louis, Missouri, March 9-13, 1986.* St Louis, Mo: CV Mosby; 1987:372-376.

59. Richards KC. Sleep promotion. *Crit Care Nurs Clin North Am.* 1996;8:39-51.

60. Richards K, Nagel C, Markie M, et al. Use of complementary and alternative therapies to promote sleep in critically ill patients. *Crit Care Nurs Clin North Am.* 2003;15(3):329-340.

61. Salamon E, Kim M, Beaulieu J, et al. Sound therapy induced relaxation: down regulating stress processes and pathologies. *Med Sci Monit.* 2003;9(5):RA116-RA121.

62. Thomas LA. Clinical management of stressors perceived by patients on mechanical ventilation. *AACN Clin Issues.* 2003;14(1):73-81.

63. Topf M, Davis JE. Critical care unit noise and rapid movement (REM) sleep. *Heart Lung.* 1993;22:252-258.

64. Tsiou C, Eftymiatos D, Theodossopoulou E, et al. Noise sources and levels in the Evgenidion Hospital intensive care unit. *Intensive Care Med.* 1998;24:845-847.

65. Walder B, Francioli D, Meyer J-J, et al. Effects of guidelines implementation in a surgical intensive care unit to control nighttime light and noise levels. *Crit Care Med.* 2000;28(7):2242-2247.

66. Wallace CJ, Robins J, Alvord LS, et al. The effect of earplugs on sleep measures during exposure to simulated intensive care unit noise. *Am J Crit Care.* 1999;8(4):210-219.

67. White JM. State of the science of music interventions. Critical care and perioperative practice. *Crit Care Nurs Clin North Am.* 2000;12(2):219-225.

68. Wilkins MK, Moore ML. Music intervention in the intensive care unit: a complementary therapy to improve patient outcomes. *Evid Based Nurs.* 2004;7(4):103-104.

69. Williamson JW. The effects of ocean sounds on sleep after coronary artery bypass graft surgery. *Am J Crit Care.* 1992;1:91-97.

70. Wong HL, Lopez-Nahas V, Molassiotis A. Effects of music therapy on anxiety in ventilator-dependent patients. *Heart Lung.* 2001;30(5):376-387.

71. Cohen RL. Art with heart in a transitional space. Dissertation Abstracts International. 1997;57(10-A):4168: 4168. University Microfilms International:1997-95007-013.

72. Marcus CC, Barnes M. *Gardens in Healthcare Facilities: Uses, Therapeutic Benefits, and Design Recommendations.* Martinez, Calif: The Center for Health Design Inc; 1995.

73. Maxion C. Art for healing. *J Health Care Interior Design.* 1989;1:85-91.

74. Roeder C. Environmental design technology: using color and light as medicine. *J Health Care Interior Design.* 1996;8:133-136.

75. Strawn J. The healing power of color. *Alt Health Pract.* 1999;5(2):173-174.

76. Ulrich RS. View through a window may influence recovery from surgery. *Science.* 1984;224:420-421.

77. Vinall PE. Design technology: what you need to know about circadian rhythms in healthcare design. *J Health Care Interior Design.* 1997;9:141-144.

78. Young-Mason J. The role of beauty, color, light and nature in the healing process. *Clin Nurs Spec.* 2002;16(4):221-222.

79. Zagon L. Selecting appropriate colors for healthcare. *J Health Care Interior Design.* 1993;5:136-141.

80. Downer K. Safety is of the essence. *Nurs Times.* 1999;95(7):14-15.

81. Dunn C, Sleep J, Collet D. Sensing an improvement: an experimental study to evaluate the use of aroma therapy, massage, and periods of rest in intensive care units. *J Adv Nurs.* 1995;21:34-40.

82. Graham PH, Browne L, Cox H, et al. Inhalation aromatherapy during radiotherapy: results of a placebo-controlled, double-blind randomized trial. *J Clin Onc.* 2003;21(12):2372-2376.

83. Merritt BA, Okyere CP, Jasinski DM. Isopropyl alcohol inhalation: alternative treatment of postoperative nausea and vomiting. *Nurs Res.* 2002;51(2):125-128.

84. Soden K, Vincent K, Craske S, et al. A randomized controlled trial of aromatherapy massage in a hospice setting. *Palliat Med.* 2004;18(2):87-92.

Family Needs, Interventions, and Presence

Jane Stover Leske, RN, PhD

Mae Ann Pasquale, RN, MSN, CCRN

Family Needs, Interventions, and Presence

CASE STUDY 1

The electronic doors of the regional trauma center's emergency entrance swung open, and Tom and Nancy Martin rushed in. Minutes earlier they had received a telephone call informing them that their 30-year-old son, Steven, had survived a head-on collision with another car and was being airlifted to the hospital. Steven's wife, Elizabeth, had been killed instantly along with the driver of the other car, which had suddenly veered into their lane of traffic.

Mr and Mrs Martin raced directly to the reception desk to ask about their son and when they could see him. Mr Martin, usually the calmer of the two parents, found himself screaming at the receptionist, who wanted to know about insurance coverage and home addresses. Those initial minutes in the waiting room seemed like hours, and the hours seemed like days. Soon, their two other children, Debra and Cynthia, joined the Martins as the emergency health care team worked vigorously to resuscitate Steven. The Martin family waited 2 hours before they received word that Steven would be transferred to the burn trauma ICU and that the next few days would determine his chances for survival.

As the family waited, several more patients were airlifted in: a man who had had a heart attack, a woman from another traffic accident, and a student who had nearly drowned were the worst of them. The admission of each patient brought other distraught family members to the waiting room. The Martin family was not alone. The sounds of acute grief reverberated throughout the waiting room.

CASE STUDY 2

The electronic doors of the regional trauma center's emergency entrance swung open, and Sam and Toni Jones rushed in. Minutes earlier they had received a telephone call informing them that their 18-year-old son, Frank, had survived a head-on collision with another car and was being airlifted to the hospital. Mr and Mrs Jones raced directly to the reception desk to ask about their son and when they could see him.

Sam and Toni received support from the moment they arrived at the hospital. A trauma support team composed of a nurse, a social worker, and a chaplain met them in the emergency department. Mr and Mrs Jones were told that Frank had a ruptured spleen, pulmonary contusions, and a compound fracture of the left femur and tibia. Although Frank's condition was critical, his parents were allowed to be present in the emergency department and to hold his hand before he was transferred to surgery.

Throughout those initial hours in the waiting room, Sam and Toni received frequent updates from the operating room nurse. When Frank was transferred to the ICU, his parents were reassured by the presence of the nurse caring for him. While Frank was in surgery, the ICU nurse and physician had introduced themselves to the Jones family and had provided explanations of what to expect in the ICU. The next 2 weeks included numerous daily concerns about infection and renal insufficiency. Throughout this time, Mr and Mrs Jones participated in Frank's care, were present on daily rounds, and were reassured that the pager the hospital provided would be used to contact them if needed whenever they were not at the hospital. Later, Frank stated that he remembered his parents' reassurances and their motivating him to fight for his life.

GENERAL DESCRIPTION

Any illness severe enough to require admission to an ICU is life threatening and can precipitate severe stress within the family system. Stresses produced by critical illness vary in intensity and duration but undeniably can create a heavy burden for families. Sources of this stress include fear of death, uncertain outcome, emotional turmoil, financial concerns, role changes, disruption of routines, and unfamiliar hospital environments. Stress may interfere with the ability of family members to receive and comprehend information, maintain patterns of family functioning, use effective coping skills, and provide positive support.

When confronted with stress, family members may experience one or more of the following: elevation in tensions, arguments, fighting among themselves, sleeplessness, feelings of helplessness, and psychosomatic manifestations. As family members struggle to cope with these stresses, the critical nature of the illness may lead to changes within the family unit. Whether these family changes are beneficial or adverse depend, in part, on the type of help the family receives from health care professionals.

Families are a unique social group involving generational ties, permanence, a concern for the total person, and a nurturing form of functioning. Originally, the term *nuclear family* referred to a family form composed of husband, wife, and children. Today the term also includes couples without children, single-parent households, reconstituted families (second marriages), unmarried couples with or without children, homosexual couples, and people living in communes. Using the traditional nuclear family form as a standard sets up a hierarchy in which some families may be valued more than others. Rather than focus on certain types of family structure, for any given critically ill patient it may be more beneficial to define a family as whoever the members of the family say they are.

In the critical care setting, families appear to have a profound beneficial impact on the critically ill patient's response to illness. Families act as buffers for patients' stress and serve as valuable resources for patients' care. However, when families have high levels of stress, they may be unable to provide support and may transfer their stress to the patient. Unmitigated family stress can manifest itself as distrust of hospital staff, noncompliance with the treatment regimen, and even lawsuits.

Because families' responses to critical illness and psychological stress have implications for the family, the patient, and the health care staff, it is advantageous for everyone to provide family-focused care so that optimal levels of family functioning are supported. Family-focused care means that nurses assess each family's needs and devise interventions to beneficially affect the outcomes of the patient and the patient's family. Nurses who support a family-focused practice model report higher autonomy and job satisfaction. The family remains the most important social context for health care professionals to positively influence patients' outcomes.

COMPETENCY

All nurses should develop competency in assessing families' needs and in intervening to address those needs. Family assessment and intervention demand expertise and theoretical knowledge. Acquiring this expertise and knowledge requires active listening and observing the interactions between patients and their family members. Nurses must have good interviewing techniques to generate family interventions in a professional manner. Some families have complex needs detected during the initial assessment. Managing hostility, anger, and great sorrow can be difficult and exhausting work. Almost all nurses benefit from education on (1) understanding the nurse-family relationship, (2) coping with situations that evolve from family interactions, and (3) improving families' satisfaction with care delivery.

ETHICAL CONSIDERATIONS

The patient and the patient's family are a unit of care, and what affects one will affect the other. Family members have a right to participate in the care of their loved one. In the era of managed care and collaboration, developing a relationship with the patient's family becomes vital to work toward the good of the patient. The issues of informed consent, advanced directives, and do-not-resuscitate orders are the most important concerns in family interventions. As care progresses and changes, ongoing discussion and negotiation are needed to confirm the patient's agreement in treatment decisions. If a family member functions as a surrogate decision maker for the patient, that member's need for information and support is as crucial as the patient's physiological needs.

SUMMARY OF CURRENT RESEARCH

Numerous studies have been done to determine the various needs of family members when one member is hospitalized in a critical care unit. Most results are based on data obtained by using the Critical Care Family Needs Inventory (CCFNI; see Appendix 2 or a modified version of this instrument). The CCFNI consists of 45 need statements that family members rate on a scale of 1 (not important) to 4 (very important). The needs have been determined in a wide range of patients, including those who had coronary disease or myocardial infarction, terminal illness, general surgery, trauma, head and spinal cord injury, burns, and cardiac surgery and general ICU populations. The results of these studies suggest that family members of critically ill patients have a well-defined predictable set of needs. These needs are grouped into 5 major areas and are universally experienced by most family members.

1. Receiving assurance—The need for assurance reflects keeping or redefining hope about the patient's outcome. Meeting this need promotes confidence, security, and freedom from doubt about the health care team and system.
2. Remaining near the patient—The need to visit reflects linking and maintaining familial relationships. Meeting this need helps family members to remain emotionally close and give support to the patient.
3. Receiving information—The need for information reflects the goal of understanding the patient's condition. Meeting this need lays the foundation for family members' decision making and coaching of the patient. Anxiety is reduced, and a sense of control is promoted.
4. Being comfortable—The need for comfort reflects reducing distress. When a person is comfortable, energy is conserved, and less stress and anxiety occur.
5. Having support available—The need for support reflects seeking or accepting expert help, assistance, or aid. Support can be physical, emotional, social, and even environmental. Meeting this need assists with coping with stress, augmenting family resources, and maintaining strength to support the patient.

Research results also show some incongruency among perceptions of patients, patients' families, and health care professionals about the importance of family needs. Family members tend to rate family needs as being more important than nurses do. Similarly, family members and nurses sometimes sharply disagree about how well family needs are met. The obvious conclusion is that developing an effective plan of care requires an assessment of the family members' perception of needs.

Much has been learned from the numerous studies that determined the importance of family members' needs after the initial impact of a critical illness. A review of the current literature indicates that sufficient descriptive research has been done on the importance of family needs. It is time to extend the results to develop and evaluate the most effective interventions for meeting these various types of family needs.

One such intervention is the Critical Care Family Assistance Program (CCFAP) developed in 2001 by the CHEST Foundation, the philanthropic arm of the American College of Chest Physicians (http://www.chestfoundation.org/Critical Care).

The CCFAP was developed to fulfill the unmet needs of the families of critically ill patients in hospital ICUs and to foster better communication between the health care team, patients, and their families. Initial results suggest that bringing together an interdisciplinary health care team to develop process, structures, and relationships with the CCFAP can facilitate satisfaction and, ultimately, positive outcomes (http://www.chestjournal.org/content/vol128/3 supp).

FUTURE RESEARCH

The literature indicates that health care professionals are placing increasing importance on the role of the patient's family during a critical illness. However, more research is needed in several areas. The following questions are proposed for further study:

- How do family needs change between the ICU phase and the rehabilitative phase?
- What are the most effective methods to promote the value of family-centered care among nurses and other health care providers?
- What organizational supports assist nurses in implementing strategies to meet the needs of patients' families?
- Which interventions best meet the family's needs in the 5 different areas of needs?
- Is it possible to predict accurately which families may be at risk for problems in adjustment?
- Can early family interventions minimize problems in adjustment?
- How do interventions reduce the physiological effects of stress?
- What is the relationship between a family's perception of nursing care quality and the family's satisfaction?
- When a patient's family is involved in care, is there a difference in the patient's outcome?
- What sensitizes nurses to families' needs, and what are the most effective ways to help nurses develop the skills needed to meet these needs?
- What is the effect of families' satisfaction on the marketing of family-centered care and on return business for the hospital?

SUGGESTED READINGS

1. Alpen MA, Halm MA. Family needs: an annotated bibliography. *Crit Care Nurse.* 1992;12(2):32, 41-50.
2. American Association of Critical-Care Nurses. Practice alert: family presence during CPR and invasive procedures. Available at: http://www.aacn.org. Accessed November 20, 2005.
3. Bahnson C. The impact of life-threatening illness on the family and the impact of the family on illness: an overview. In: Leahey M, Wright LM, eds. *Families and Life-Threatening Illness.* Springhouse, Pa: Springhouse; 1987:26-44.
4. Danielson CB, Hamel-Bissell B, Winstead-Fry P, eds. *Families, Health, and Illness: Perspectives on Coping and Intervention.* St. Louis, Mo: CV Mosby; 1993.
5. Denham S. *Family Health: A Framework for Nursing.* Philadelphia, Pa: FA Davis; 2003.
6. Feetham SL, Meister SB, Bell JM, Gilliss CL, eds. *The Nursing of Families: Theory/Research/Education/Practice.* Newbury Park, Calif: Sage; 1993.
7. Friedman MM, Bowden VR, Jones EJ. *Family Nursing:*

Research, Theory, and Practice. Pearson Education: Prentice Hall; 2003.

8. Halm MA. Family presence during resuscitation: a critical review of the literature. *Am J Crit Care*. 2005;14:494-511.

9. Halm MA, Titler MG, Kleiber C, et al. Behavioral responses of family members during critical illness. *Clin Nurs Res*. 1993;2:414-437.

10. Leske JS. Needs of adult family members after critical illness. *Crit Care Nurs Clin North Am*. 1992;4:587-596.

11. Leske JS. Comparison ratings of need importance after critical illness from family members with varied demographic characteristics. *Crit Care Nurs Clin North Am*. 1992;4:607-613.

12. Leske JS, Vaughan-Cole B, O'Neill-Conger C, et al. Interviewing the family unit. In: Vaughan-Cole B, Johnson MA, Malone JA, et al, eds. *Family Nursing Practice*. Philadelphia, Pa: Saunders; 1998:61-74.

13. McCubbin HI, Thompson EA, Thompson AI, et al, eds. *Stress, Coping, and Health in Families: Sense of Coherence and Resiliency*. Thousand Oaks, Calif: Sage; 1998.

14. McKenry PC, Price S. *Families and Change: Coping with Stressful Events and Transitions*. Thousand Oaks, Calif: Sage; 2000.

15. Whall AL, Fawcett J. *Family Theory Development in Nursing: State of the Science and Art*. Philadelphia, Pa: FA Davis; 1991.

16. White JM, Klein DM, eds. *Family Theories*. Thousand Oaks, Calif: Sage; 2002.

17. Wright LM, Leahey M, eds. *Nurses and Families: A Guide to Family Assessment and Intervention*. Philadelphia, Pa: FA Davis; 2005.

CLINICAL RECOMMENDATIONS

The rating scale for the Level of Recommendation ranges from I to VI, with levels indicated as follows: I, manufacturer's recommendations only; II, theory based, no research data to support recommendations; recommendations from expert consensus group may exist; III, laboratory data only, no clinical data to support recommendations; IV, limited clinical studies to support recommendations; V, clinical studies in more than 1 or 2 different populations and situations to support recommendations; VI, clinical studies in a variety of patient populations and situations to support recommendations.

Family Needs

Period of Use	Recommendation	Rationale for Recommendation	Level of Recommendation	Supporting References	Comments
Selection of Patients	Adult family members of patients who are admitted to critical care		VI: Clinical studies in a variety of populations and situations	See Annotated Bibliography: 3 See Other References: 2, 16, 25, 26, 35, 43, 59, 63, 65, 66, 75, 76, 80, 84, 91, 95, 99, 100, 113, 116, 121, 168, 191, 278, 281, 283, 287, 297	Parents of critically ill children are also included.
Application and Use	Providing family-focused care involves 4 steps: assessment, planning, intervention, and evaluation.	Some reliable and valid family assessment tools are available	VI: Clinical studies in a variety of populations and situations	See Other References: 15, 78, 84, 97, 146	
	Assessment				
	Initiate family contact early. Include the following: • Instill realistic hope. • Answer questions honestly. • Assure the family that the best care possible is being given.	Early contact fosters a trusting relationship Promotes family satisfaction.	VI: Clinical studies in a variety of populations and situations	See Suggested Readings: 9, 10 See Annotated Bibliography: 3 See Other References: 11, 16, 17, 21, 25, 26, 41, 43, 45, 46, 50, 52, 54, 56, 58, 59, 62, 80, 81, 89, 96, 99, 100, 113, 116, 121, 145, 190, 206, 218, 285, 287, 300, 301	
	Start a family assessment database:	A database lays the foundation for planning and helps align expectations with interventions to promote satisfaction.	VI: Clinical studies in a variety of populations and situations	See Suggested Readings: 3-5, 9, 15 See Other References: 9, 13, 14, 22, 24, 29, 36, 37, 46, 47, 55, 74, 86, 87, 98, 114, 115, 128, 145, 203, 208, 218, 228, 279, 284, 286, 289, 300	See the appendix for the CCFNI.
	• Use open-ended communication. • Assess family members' level of anxiety. • Assess family members' perception of the situation.	Family anxiety may influence patient anxiety. Family perception may affect patient perception.			

Period of Use	Recommendation	Rationale for Recommendation	Level of Recommendation	Supporting References	Comments
Application and Use (*cont.*)	*Assessment (cont.)*				
	• Assess family roles and dynamics.	Families search for meaning and hope in the present situation.			
	• Assess family members' coping mechanisms and resources.	Family resources also include knowledge, health, decision-making skills, and interfamily support.			
	Explore family strengths and reinforce them.	Family strengths are a catalyst for healthy family functioning.	IV: Limited clinical studies to support recommendations	See Other References: 15, 46, 154, 203, 213, 218	
	Assess family developmental stage.	Family developmental stage influences family functioning.			
	Explore family structure and home environment.	There may be other family members who are affected by the illness.			
	Explore family culture.	Each family has a unique set of values and beliefs.			
	Assess family support network.	Quality of support has been reported to be crucial to patient well-being and family adaptation.			
	Planning				
	Determine what the family needs most at this time.	It is best to begin at the family's level.	IV: Limited clinical studies to support recommendations	See Suggested Readings: 3, 9, 10, 15 See Other References: 4, 8, 10, 12, 13, 15, 23, 26, 33, 40, 120, 161, 218	
	Determine if other health care professionals should be consulted.	Involving other health care professionals reduces the frustration of ICU staff members and gives ICU personnel more time to care for other patients.			
	Use care conferences or daily contact to include family members in planning care.	Care conferences give families the opportunity to participate.			
	Start a discharge plan.				
	Interventions				
	Determine who will act as the family's spokesperson and support persons.	Having a family spokesperson provides continuity.	VI: Clinical studies in a variety of populations and situations	See Suggested Readings: 4, 9, 10, 15 See Other References: 15, 25, 26, 38, 46, 60, 92, 99, 117, 121, 129, 134-136, 137, 139, 142, 143, 145, 152, 154, 157, 159, 160, 167, 168, 171, 177,	

Period of Use	Recommendation	Rationale for Recommendation	Level of Recommendation	Supporting References	Comments
Application and Use (*cont.*)	*Interventions (cont.)*			181, 218, 280, 287, 295, 297, 301	
	Determine who will be the contact person for the family.	Having a contact person helps the family understand the patient's condition and assists in discharge.			
	Establish the mechanism for family members' access to the patient:				
	• Open visitation				
	• Contract visitation				
	• Specific rules: any adjustments needed?				
	• Unit telephone numbers				
	Promote access to patients by having unit policies to ensure continuity among staff members.				
	Offer a tour of the ICU.		VI: Clinical studies in a variety of populations and situations	See Other References: 5, 15, 16, 26, 30-32, 34, 38, 39, 42, 54, 58, 60, 64, 66, 80, 81, 92, 94, 99, 101, 105, 115, 125, 126, 128, 129, 133-135, 137, 138, 139, 141, 142, 145, 156, 159, 162, 166, 174, 175, 180, 218, 277, 281, 283, 284, 287-292, 294-296	
	Establish a mechanism to contact the family:				
	• Telephone numbers				
	• Beeper system				
	Provide consistent information according to the family's needs:	It has been reported that providing consistent information and allowing sufficient time for giving information are two predictors of family satisfaction.	VI: Clinical studies in a variety of populations and situations	See Suggested Readings: 1, 9 See Other References: 26, 52, 68, 80, 92, 117, 124, 292, 297, 299, 300	
	• Care conferences				
	• Videotapes				
	• Audiotapes				
	• Information booklets				
	• Attendance at bedside rounds				
	• Support groups	Support groups unite families with similar concerns and experiences.	VI: Clinical studies in a variety of populations and situations	See Annotated Bibliography 2 See Other References: 52, 127, 141, 142, 164, 173, 294, 301	
	Act as an advocate to connect family members with the patient's physicians.				
	Ensure that support services are available.				

Period of Use	Recommendation	Rationale for Recommendation	Level of Recommendation	Supporting References	Comments
Application and Use (*cont.*)	*Interventions (cont.)* Explain all procedures in understandable terms.				
	Encourage family to discuss any problems.	This improves psychosocial family adjustment.			
	Include the family in providing direct care to the patient: • Have them help the patient with activities of daily living. • Have them provide diversion with audiotapes, videotapes, music, pictures, story reading, and so forth. • Have them assist with care activities as appropriate.	Certain cultures show their concerns and feeling for each other by taking care of the patient's physical needs.	VI: Clinical studies in a variety of populations and situations	See Other References: 15, 83, 85, 218, 123, 223	
	Include family members in end-of-life planning and implementation.	Changes in patient prognosis will affect the type of family intervention needed.	VI: Clinical studies in a variety of populations and situations	See Annotated Bibliography 6 See Other References: 20, 105, 135, 149, 220, 221, 222, 225, 228, 229, 230, 231, 232, 293, 306	
	Provide palliative care and support for terminally ill patients and the patients' families.	The attitude of the health care professional is one of the most important aspects of giving bad news.			
	Provide a comfortable environment for the family. • Comfortable furniture • Volunteer support in the waiting area • Quiet room available • Easy access to telephones and rest rooms • Arranging for accommodations for family members from out of town • Allow time for family to be alone		VI: Clinical studies in a variety of populations and situations	See Annotated Bibliography: 1, 2, 3 See Other References: 16, 26, 51, 58, 59, 66, 80, 83, 84, 91, 95, 100, 116, 287, 302	
	• Encourage family members to take care of themselves	Complementary and alternative therapies may promote sleep and reduce stress.	IV: Limited clinical studies	See Other References: 146	

Period of Use	Recommendation	Rationale for Recommendation	Level of Recommendation	Supporting References	Comments
Application and Use (*cont.*)	*Interventions (cont.)* Establish a system such as daily communication to update the family on changes in the patient's condition.	The need for information has emerged as the most important family need.	VI: Clinical studies in a variety of populations and situations	See Annotated Bibliography 3 See Other References: 2, 5, 15, 16, 19, 26, 53, 56, 58, 80, 100, 103, 116, 218, 281, 283, 287, 290, 299	
	Refer family members to specialized support services as needed (eg, chaplain, social worker, financial officer, clinical nurse specialist, support group).		IV: Limited clinical studies	See Other References: 7, 155, 218, 305	
	Be alert to dysfunctional family adaptation and immediately refer to the advanced practice nurse.	It may be useful for the Advanced Practice Nurse to use The Synergy Model to help guide families.			
	Evaluation Evaluate family members' responses to interventions by using a variety of mechanisms: • Feedback in support groups		VI: Clinical studies in a variety of populations and situations	See Other References: 15, 125, 145, 167, 182, 183, 185, 187, 188, 189-191, 193, 219, 227, 232, 280, 282, 290, 293, 298, 303, 304	
	• Family satisfaction surveys	Family dissatisfaction can occur anytime while the patient is in the critical care unit.		See Other References: 186, 188, 193, 218	
	• Family-to-staff communication book in the waiting area	Family satisfaction questionnaires are available.			
	• Multidisciplinary conferences with family members • Individual communication with family members	Nurses and physicians have underestimated the family's need for information.	VI: Clinical studies in a variety of populations and situations	See Annotated Bibliography: 3 See Other References: 17, 53, 82, 107, 155, 195, 205, 287	
	• Interdisciplinary rounds • Weekly discharge planning conferences	Allows all disciplines to participate in patient/family outcomes, early recognition of patient at risk, and improved communication among members of the health care team.			
	• Follow-up after discharge	Caregivers may experience substantial burden due to the complexity of the patient's treatment and functional ability.		See Other References: 150, 165, 197, 198, 207, 215, 216, 218, 296, 298	

Period of Use	Recommendation	Rationale for Recommendation	Level of Recommendation	Supporting References	Comments
Ongoing Monitoring	Use the evaluation mechanisms listed in the previous section. Observe family members' responses.		VI: Clinical studies in a variety of populations and situations	See Other References: 79, 120, 145, 167, 184, 189-191, 280, 282, 290, 293, 296, 298	
	Assess the potential of transfer stress by asking both patient and family. Develop standardized ICU transfer protocols and teaching programs.	Patients and family members perceive transfer from the ICU as a significant and sometimes negative event.	VI: Clinical studies in a variety of populations and situations	See Other References: 150, 165, 170, 206, 211, 212, 214	
Quality Control Issues	Provide ongoing in-service training to professional staff.	Special knowledge and skills are needed to deliver family care in a sensitive and compassionate manner.	V: Clinical studies in more than 1 or 2 different populations or situations	See Other References: 15, 44, 61, 64, 71, 79, 96, 103, 170, 183, 186, 189, 191, 197, 202	Perceived staff competency is of great significance to family members. Providing a family-centered approach in critical care requires advanced skill.
	Develop conflict resolution process and policies. Understand Patient Bill of Rights. Use health care directives as a guide for the treatment plan.				
	Use continuous quality improvement as a framework to gather family responses to the critical care experience.	Quality improvement projects are necessary to reduce the gap between family needs and satisfaction levels.			

Family Presence

Period of Use	Recommendation	Rationale for Recommendation	Level of Recommendation	Supporting References	Comments
Selection of Patients	Adult family members of patients who are critically ill or injured		V: Clinical studies in more than 1 or 2 different populations and situations	See Other References: 236, 237, 238, 241, 252, 256, 259, 261, 269, 308, 310, 312	Parents of critically ill and injured children are also included.
Application and Use	Providing the option for family to be present for invasive procedures (IP) and/or resuscitation involves 4 steps: assessment, planning, intervention, and evaluation.	Family-centered care provides the framework for providing the option for family presence during IP and resuscitation events. Emergency care requires assessment and intervention to meet the patient's and family's full spectrum of needs.	VI: Clinical studies in a variety of populations or situations	See Suggested Readings: 2 See Other References: 233, 234, 236, 237, 238, 239, 242, 244, 247, 248, 249, 252, 254, 256, 257, 259, 261, 271, 272, 308, 310, 312	

Period of Use	Recommendation	Rationale for Recommendation	Level of Recommendation	Supporting References	Comments
Application and Use (*cont.*)	*Assessment* Initiate family contact early. Include the following: • Instill a realistic, yet hopeful perception of the situation. • Answer questions honestly. • Assure the family that the best possible care is being provided.	Early family involvement is essential to meet the patient's and family's psychosocial, emotional, and spiritual needs, as well as physical needs. Family members fear that health care providers will withhold information about their loved ones. Families in crisis need reassurance and informational support to cope effectively.	VI: Clinical studies in a variety of populations or situations	See Annotated Bibliography: 3 See Suggested Readings: 2 See Other References: 16, 17, 26, 41, 54, 80, 81, 100, 108, 109, 110, 235, 236, 237, 238, 241, 244, 245, 247, 254, 259, 265, 269, 274, 275, 287, 301, 310, 311	
	Assess the patient's and family's desires and needs to be present during IP and/or resuscitation as soon as possible.	Exclusion of the family from the treatment area, when they want to be with their loved one, can perpetuate feelings of helplessness and being uninvolved.	V: Clinical studies in more than 1 or 2 different populations and situations	See Annotated Bibliography: 3 See Suggested Readings: 2 See Other References: 14, 46, 74, 86, 98, 130, 145, 146, 203, 218, 235, 236, 238, 247, 248, 256, 259, 271, 274, 279, 300, 308, 310, 312	Initially, if the patient can communicate, it is important to determine their preference about having a family member present. In most cases, the patient will be unconscious and so this will not be possible.
	• Use focused questions to elicit information about the patient's and/or family's perception of the situation.	Family members feel a need to be close to and protect the patients when threatened by the permanent loss of their loved ones.			
	• Assess the patient's and/or family's willingness and comfort with being present.	Family members who remain at the bedside during resuscitative attempts view themselves as "active participants" in the care of the patient.			
	• Assess the patient's and/or family's previous experiences.	Identifying the patient's and family's understanding of and reaction to the critical situation as well as previous coping mechanisms provides a foundation for further interaction and intervention.			
	• Assess family member's level of anxiety. • Assess the family's customary coping strategies.	Screening of family members is necessary to prevent those who are believed not to be able to cope from being further traumatized. The option to			

Period of Use	Recommendation	Rationale for Recommendation	Level of Recommendation	Supporting References	Comments
Application and Use (*cont.*)	*Assessment (cont.)*	visit should be conditional, based on the family's emotional and physical tolerance of the situation.			
	Explore the family's established support systems.	The availability of a health professional to offer support is important to families.	IV: Limited clinical studies to support recommendations	See Other References: 60, 74, 83, 85, 114, 178, 203, 218, 247, 254	
		Quality of support is crucial to patient well-being and family adaptation.			
	Assess the family's culture, lifestyle, and customs.	The customs and practices of individual families influence the way they communicate (verbal and nonverbal), make decisions, grieve, and adapt to crisis-producing events.			
	Assess the family's ability to express their needs.	It is very important that family presence remains an option and does not turn into an emotional obligation.	V: Clinical studies in more than 1 or 2 different populations and situations	See Suggested Readings: 2 See Other References: 233, 241, 246, 247, 249, 259, 268, 271, 274, 275, 307, 310	
	Be supportive and unbiased of patients who choose not to have family members present and family members who choose not to be present during such events.	Family members could perceive that they are doing something wrong when they do not attend the resuscitative effort.	V: Clinical studies in more than 1 or 2 different populations and situations	See Suggested Readings: 2 See Other References: 233, 236, 237, 238, 239, 241, 242, 243, 245, 247, 248, 249, 252, 256, 258, 259, 269, 271, 275, 310, 311	
	Planning				
	Inform the direct care providers (physicians and nurses) of the family's arrival and request to be present for the IP or resuscitation.	The decision to have the family present in the treatment room depends on the family's desire to be present and the agreement of the direct care providers.		Suggested Readings: 2	
	Determine the patient and family's support needs.	It is reported that the quality of the interaction between the health care providers and the family is a significant factor in how the family views the experience.			
	Determine who will act as the family spokesperson.	Having a family spokesperson provides continuity.			

Period of Use	Recommendation	Rationale for Recommendation	Level of Recommendation	Supporting References	Comments
Application and Use (*cont.*)	*Planning (cont.)* Determine who will act in the family support person role.	A knowledgeable trained staff member, which may include nurses, physicians, chaplains, social workers, and other trained personnel, must be identified to function in the family support person role.			
	Determine the process needed to bring the family to the bedside as soon as possible, if only briefly.	Although there may be specific circumstances that are restrictive, it is no longer acceptable to routinely keep families outside of the treatment area.	V: Clinical studies in more than 1 or 2 different populations and situations	Suggested Reading: 2 See Other References: 15, 25, 38, 46, 60, 92, 117, 121, 137, 152, 241, 242, 244, 247, 252, 254, 258, 259, 271, 272, 275, 297, 300, 307	
	Interventions Initiate involvement of the family support person as soon as the need is identified.	The purpose of the family support person is to maintain an awareness of the patient's and family's psychosocial and emotional needs and to initiate interventions to assist in meeting those needs.	IV: Limited clinical studies to support recommendations	See Suggested Readings: 2 See Other References: 242, 245, 247, 248, 252, 272, 275	
	Clearly inform the family of the status of the patient. Provide the family timely information concerning the performance of procedures and other interventions. Explain all procedures and equipment in understandable terms, avoiding medical jargon.	Receiving information, understanding the care and procedures provided, providing comfort, and being comforted are the most important family needs during critical events.	V: Clinical studies in more than 1 or 2 different populations and situations	See Other References: 240, 241, 246, 247, 249, 250, 251, 252, 253, 255, 258, 259, 260, 265, 273, 307, 309, 310	
	Describe the sights, sounds, and smells that may be encountered by the family member in the resuscitation area. Describe to the family potential responses that the patient may exhibit to the family member. Emphasize to the family that patient care is the priority.	Preparing the family member, psychologically and cognitively, before they enter the resuscitation area will enhance their coping ability of the situation.	VI: Clinical studies in a variety of populations or situations	See Other References: 26, 68, 80, 92, 117, 163, 247, 275, 297, 299	

Period of Use	Recommendation	Rationale for Recommendation	Level of Recommendation	Supporting References	Comments
Application and Use (*cont.*)	*Interventions (cont.)* Clarify the family member's role in providing comfort and reassurance to the patient.				
	Establish the process for family member access to the patient: • How many family members will enter the room at one time? • Where will the family members stand initially? • When can the family member move to the bedside?	Setting limits and communicating information concerning the process of entering and exiting the resuscitation area can provide valuable guidance to the family members.	V: Clinical studies in more than 1 or 2 different populations and situations	See Other References: 129, 140, 242, 244, 245, 247, 249, 254, 258, 261, 263, 272, 275	
	Explain to the family that if they exhibit any uncontrolled outbursts, violent behavior, etc., they will be restricted from the bedside at that time.	Individuals acting hysterically, demonstrating aggressive behavior, or showing signs of an altered mental status should not be allowed into the resuscitation room as they could interfere with the emergency procedure, thus putting the patient at risk, as well as causing possible long-term psychological damage to themselves.			
	Accompany the family to the bedside: • Verbally advise all direct care providers that the family is present.	The attitudes of health care providers affect the family member's decision to stay or leave the room.	VI: Clinical studies in a variety of populations or situations	See Annotated Bibliography: 1, 2, 3 See Other References: 16, 26, 51, 58, 59, 66, 80, 83, 84, 91, 95, 100, 116, 287, 302	
	• Provide explanations of the interventions initiated and interpret medical jargon. • Provide information concerning the patient's response to treatments and expected outcomes. • Use terminology appropriate to the person's level of understanding.	Preparing the family includes readying the individuals for all invasive procedures in a manner that reflects consideration of the patient's developmental level and the family member's level of understanding.	IV: Limited clinical studies to support recommendations	See Suggested Readings: 2 See Other References: 238, 243, 247, 256, 267, 273, 311	

Period of Use	Recommendation	Rationale for Recommendation	Level of Recommendation	Supporting References	Comments
Application and Use (*cont.*)	*Interventions (cont.)*				
	• Assess the family member's understanding of the information.	Due to the critical nature of the situation, family members may not always comprehend the information the first time it is provided.			
	• Provide opportunities for questions and clarify the details.	Clinical information may need to be repeated or restated several times prior to comprehension.			
	• Role model supportive and enduring behaviors.	When family members are present, nurses' interactions should go beyond providing information toward supporting enduring behaviors among both patients and patient's family members.			
	• Provide opportunities for the family member to touch and speak to the patient.	It is important that the family member knows that the patient may be able to hear.			
	Never leave a family member unattended at the bedside during resuscitative events or invasive procedures.	The primary responsibility of the family support person is to stay with the family member and to provide emotional support.	VI: Clinical studies in a variety of populations or situations	See Other References: 15, 125, 145, 183, 185, 188, 189, 190, 191, 193, 219, 227, 232, 238, 241, 243, 247, 252, 256, 257, 280, 298, 303, 310, 311	
	Provide privacy for patient and family member if possible.				
	If intrahospital transport for procedures is needed, provide the family with a comfortable waiting environment:	Refer to Environmental Design and Strategies to Promote Healing (Chapter 1) Clinical Recommendations			
	• Comfortable furniture				
	• Volunteer support in the waiting area				
	• Quiet room available				
	• Easy access to telephones and restrooms				
	Assist with accommodations for family members that are arriving from out of town.				

Period of Use	Recommendation	Rationale for Recommendation	Level of Recommendation	Supporting References	Comments
Application and Use (*cont.*)	*Interventions (cont.)*				
	Promote access to the patient care unit as soon as the patient is admitted.	Faced with potential death and disability, the immense benefits of family presence for family members include knowing that everything was done for the patient, feeling that they had supported the patient, reducing family anxiety and fear, and easing their bereavement.			
	If death has occurred:				
	• Inform family of death in clear language.				
	• Explain that everything possible was done.				
	• Work with the family support person to facilitate the family's viewing of the body, requests for tissue/ organ donation, and requests for autopsy.				
	• Allow the family as much time to stay with the deceased family member.	Family presence provides a sense of closure on a life shared together.			
	• Offer family bereavement follow-up, if needed.	Bereavement follow-up programs have been implemented in many hospitals to facilitate continued family assessment and intervention/referral.			
	Evaluation				
	Evaluate the family members' responses to interventions by using a variety of mechanisms:	Follow-up contact provides the family an opportunity to ask questions, seek additional information, discuss or review concerns, and validate those interventions that were effective or helpful and those that were not.	V: Clinical studies in more than 1 or 2 different populations and situations	See Other References: 242, 245, 247, 249, 250, 252, 265, 268, 271, 275, 309, 310	
	• Feedback in support groups				
	• Family satisfaction surveys				
	• Individual communication with family members				
	Follow-up with telephone calls or correspondence as appropriate.	Follow-up interaction with the family affords the staff an opportunity to further assess the psychosocial needs of the family.			
	Evaluate the staff's responses to interventions and need for support services.	The timing of the follow-up evaluation should be considered in relation to the clinical situation and outcome.			

Period of Use	Recommendation	Rationale for Recommendation	Level of Recommendation	Supporting References	Comments
Application and Use (*cont.*)	*Evaluation (cont.)*				
	Encourage staff to talk about their experiences and feelings at team meetings and educational sessions.	Any resuscitation can be stressful to the staff. The presence of family members during IP or resuscitation is often emotionally challenging for staff.			
		Staff who practice in acute care settings have developed personal strategies to cope with the stressors and emotional demands of their work environments. There are times, however, when their usual coping strategies may be surpassed.			
	Offer hospital- or community-based critical incident stress management (CISM) for debriefing and defusing of events within 24 to 72 hours of the event.	CISM programs help to speed recovery and assist staff with decreasing the negative after-effects of resuscitation.			
	Encourage the use of Employee Assistance Programs for managing individual stress.				
Ongoing Monitoring	Use the evaluation mechanisms listed in the previous section.	Family members need to be evaluated regarding the long-term effects of viewing the resuscitation.	VI: Clinical studies in a variety of populations or situations	See Other References: 15, 125, 145, 184, 189, 190, 191, 227, 238, 247, 256, 257, 303, 310, 311	
	Observe family members' responses to being present.				
	Continually assess the Family Presence policy and procedural processes.				
Quality Control Issues	Provide open forums for the multidisciplinary staff to discuss attitudes, concerns, and beliefs regarding family presence.	Health care providers often express fear that family members will increase the stress of the resuscitation team and disrupt medical procedures. Family members are also viewed as a possible source of legal liability.	IV: Limited clinical studies to support recommendations	See Other References: 235, 239, 240, 242, 246, 247, 250, 253, 260, 265, 271, 275, 309	
	Survey/interview the professional and administrative staff to identify current practices and potential barriers.	Providing opportunities for staff expression allows concerns and potential roadblocks to be addressed. Examining the operating procedures and policies related to			

Period of Use	Recommendation	Rationale for Recommendation	Level of Recommendation	Supporting References	Comments
Quality Control Issues (*cont.*)		family presence provides information about the current organization- and department-based practices.			
	Develop strategies to increase awareness and to gain acceptance of this practice: • Post family presence articles on the unit. • Conduct informal and formal educational presentations. • Hold clinical/ethics conferences. • Journal clubs • Case presentations	Strategies that raise the consciousness of the staff and addresses staff concerns is a necessity for changing the mind-set and attitudes of the staff. Education can change nurses' beliefs regarding the presence of family members in the resuscitation room.	IV: Limited clinical studies to support recommendations	See Suggested Readings: 2 See Other References: 44, 202, 234, 235, 242, 245, 247, 249, 254, 259, 271, 272, 275, 307, 309	
	Solicit and share family and health care provider experiences of family presence.	Studies have shown that health care providers with previous experience with family presence are more likely to support this practice.			
	Conduct a needs assessment and provide ongoing educational sessions to the professional staff.	Education of staff provides the skills needed to support families during IP and resuscitation and is an important component in both promoting family-centered care and changing practice to support family presence.			
	Use the Emergency Nurses Association's (ENA) "Presenting the Option for Family Presence" guideline as a resource for a family presence policy and educational program. Use the AACN Practice Alert, *Family Presence During CPR and Invasive Procedures,* to assist in educating administration and staff about the evidence to support this practice.	The ENA and AACN believe it is in the best interest of the patient and family to offer the option for a family member to be present during invasive procedures and resuscitation situations. This belief is endorsed through the ENA's position statement and FP guideline and the AACN Practice Alert related to this subject.			

ANNOTATED BIBLIOGRAPHY

Family Assessment

1. Bournes DA, Mitchell GJ. Waiting: The experience of persons in a critical care waiting room. *Res Nurs Health*. 2002;25:58-67.

Study Sample

A convenience sample of 10 women and 2 men agreed to speak to the researchers about their experience of waiting.

Comparison Studied

The study examined the experiences of waiting for persons who have family members in a critical care unit. The findings were to provide information about what it is like to wait in order to guide practice and research.

Study Procedures

Parse's phenomenological-hermeneutic method was used. The researcher asked family members to "please tell me about your experience of waiting." The dialogue was audiotaped and transcribed verbatim.

Key Results

Three core concepts were extracted and synthesized from the interview data. These concepts were vigilant attentiveness, ambiguous turbulent lull, and contentment with uplifting engagements. Vigilant attentiveness was a focused, persistent, and diligent watchfulness. A grueling experience of unsure stillness captured the ambiguous turbulent lull. Contentment with uplifting engagements described the calming and comforting experiences of helpful associations with others in the waiting room.

Study Strengths and Weaknesses

Enhancing understanding about what it is like to wait would be helpful to health care professionals. The 3 core concepts ought to lead to further research. Qualitative findings are difficult to replicate.

Clinical Implications

The findings may help nurses: (1) listen to the experiences of waiting, (2) have a better understanding of the waiting experience, and (3) respect the wishes of the family to be near their loved one. It is important to encourage family interaction in the waiting room. Several units have instituted a family waiting room "group." The purpose of the group is to listen to the experiences of family members.

2. DeJong MJ, Beatty DS. Family perceptions of support interventions in the intensive care unit. *Dimens Crit Care Nurs*. 2000;19:40-47.

Study Sample

The convenience sample consisted of 84 family members of critically ill patients. Most family members reported they were the spouse (63%) and Caucasian (66%).

Comparison Studied

The study examined family perceptions regarding the importance of support interventions and the frequency with which the nursing staff provided those interventions.

Study Procedures

Family members were asked to participate 24 to 48 hours after patient admission to ICU. Participants completed a self-report tool, which included information about visitation. In addition, information was obtained about 12 specific types of assistance offered at the facility.

Key Results

Results indicated 4 areas of support. These areas were: information/communication support, appraisal support, emotional support, and instrumental support. The family members considered informational support the most important. The same interventions that families considered most important also were those that nurses provided the most often.

Study Strengths and Weaknesses

The major limitations were the small sample size and the amount of missing data. The majority of participants did not complete the section that asked about specific interventions particular to the setting.

Clinical Implication

Several supportive interventions are identified in this study. The most important interventions for this study's sample were: notifying the family about changes in the patient's condition, answering the family's questions, explaining everything being done for the patient, and allowing the family to visit as much as desired. Other recommendations were to include the family in patient care, arrange a family care conference, assess family coping, promote family-centered care, and refer the family as needed.

3. Leske JS. Needs of family members after critical illness: prescriptions for interventions. *Crit Care Nurs Clin North Am*. 1992;4:587-596.

Study Sample

The integrated sample included 905 family members of 668 critically ill patients.

Comparison Studied

The results of several research studies on the needs of family members of the critically ill are summarized.

Study Procedures

Data from 27 researchers, in 15 states, over a period of 10 years (1980-1989), and in 38 different critical care units were combined. Studies that used the CCFNI and collected data from family members in the first 72 hours of the patient's admission to critical care were accepted for analysis. Factor analysis was used to organize the 5 need categories on the CCFNI.

Key Results

The 5 need categories are labeled as assurance, proximity, information, comfort, and support. Assurance reflects the family's need to hope for a desired outcome, part of which is based on their confidence and trust in the health care team. Proximity mirrors the family members' needs for personal contact and to be physically and emotionally near the critically ill person. After initial notification of a critical illness, all families need to have consistent and realistic information about their ill member. Personal comforts allow family members to remain near the ill members for longer periods. Support reflects the variety of resources, support systems, or supportive structures that families need after a critical illness.

Study Strengths and Weaknesses

The findings support the results of previous studies.

Clinical Implications

Research results consistently suggest that families of critically ill patients place the utmost importance on receiving assurance about the treatment and prognosis of the patient, remaining near the patient, receiving information about the condition of the patient, having environmental comforts, and receiving support from health care personnel. These need categories provided the context for designing and testing interventions for meeting the needs of patients' family members.

Family Interventions

4. **Johnson KL, Cheung RB, Johnson SB, et al. Therapeutic paralysis of critically ill trauma patients: perceptions of patients and their family members.** *Am J Crit Care*. 1999;7:490-498.

Study Sample

Eleven pairs of subjects participated in the study. Each pair consisted of one critically ill adult trauma patient and one member of the patient's family.

Comparison Studied

The purpose of the study was to obtain the recollections of therapeutic paralysis in critically ill trauma patients and to determine the psychological, emotional, and educational needs of patients' family members during the time the patient was paralyzed.

Study Procedures

A qualitative phenomenological approach was used to investigate the lived experience of the patient and family member during therapeutic paralysis. Each patient and his or her family member were interviewed on the same occasion after discharge from the ICU. A semistructured interview guide was used to describe the experiences and needs of patients and family members during therapeutic paralysis.

Key Results

Patients recalled their experience of therapeutic paralysis with vagueness, as if they had been dreaming. Few recalled pain or painful procedures. Patients remember nurse and family members providing emotional support and encouragement. Family members remembered being encouraged to touch and talk to the patient.

Study Strengths and Weaknesses

Generalizability is limited due to the small sample size and qualitative methods.

Clinical Implications

It appears that pain and sedation protocols used in conjunction with therapeutic paralysis are effective in suppressing patients' awareness of unpleasant events. Patients appear to not specifically recall being paralyzed. It is important for nurses to work with those who will remember the experience: the family members. Family members can provide the patient with the encouragement that is needed for optimal recovery. It is important to teach family members about the therapeutic paralysis and events that occur when the paralysis is being reversed.

Evaluation of Family Outcomes

5. **Swoboda SM, Lipsett PA. Impact of a prolonged surgical critical illness on patients' families.** *Am J Crit Care*. 2002;11:459-466.

Study Sample

A total of 128 patients met the entry criteria, and families of surviving patients were interviewed at baseline and 1, 3, 6, and 12 months later.

Comparison Studied

The purpose of this study was to determine the impact of the patients' illness on family caregiving and lifestyle alteration. It was hypothesized that prolonged illness would have a long-lasting effect of patients' families that would be related to patients' functional outcomes.

Study Procedures

Family members of all patients staying for more than 6 days in the ICU were asked to participate. Patients' quality of life was measured. The effects of insurance status on baseline family demographics, family caregiving, and financial burdens also were examined.

Key Results

Significant disturbances in the family's lives occurred throughout the 12 months of this study. Almost 60% of responding families provided a moderate or large amount of caregiving between 1 and 9 months after a prolonged illness, 45% had to quit work after one month, and more than 36% lost savings after one year. Some families moved to a less expensive home, delayed educational plans, or delayed medical care for another family member.

Study Strengths and Weaknesses

These findings are supported by several other studies. None of the families in this study had private insurance, which would have influenced the results related to financial loss. Families of patients who died were not interviewed. The family burden after death needs to be determined in further research.

Clinical Implications

An acute illness that has a prolonged stay in an ICU has a substantial effect on patients' family members that is maximal between 1 and 3 months after discharge. This burden parallels the patient's functional status. There needs to be continued assessment after ICU discharge of the patient's illness and the impact of that illness on the family.

End-of-Life Care

6. **Ahrens T, Yancey V, Kollef M. Improving family communications at the end-of-life: implications for length of stay in the intensive care unit and resource use.** *Am J Crit Care.* **2003;12:317-324.**

Study Sample

During a 1-year period, patients deemed to be at high risk for dying were divided into 2 groups: 108 patients in the standard practice or control group who received care by an attending physician and 43 patients who were cared for by the medical director teamed with a clinical nurse specialist (CNS) as the intervention group.

Comparison Studied

This quality improvement project evaluated the effect of a physician-nurse communication team to improve opportunities for patients and their families to discuss medical information and effective treatments. Measured patient outcomes included length of stay and costs for patients near the end of life in the intensive care unit.

Study Procedures

To improve the performance of the communication team, barriers to effective communication with families of seri-

ously ill patients in ICU were identified. Specific roles for the physician and the CNS were defined to address the barriers. Physicians provided daily medical updates to patients' families, offered guidelines for care, and shared medical advice concerning treatment options. The CNS provided daily information to families, allowed time for discussion and interpretation, and reinforced the medical treatment plan.

Key Results

When families had consistent communication with the physician-CNS team, patients had shorter hospital stays and reduced costs. The average ICU length of stay was reduced from 9.5 days in the standard practice group to 6.1 days in the intervention group. The overall hospital stay also was significantly reduced in the intervention group. In addition, hospital direct and indirect costs were lower in the intervention group.

Study Strengths and Weaknesses

Quality improvement projects lack the rigor of research. The education efforts in this study focused on one physician and the CNS. Whether another nurse with skill in communication could have the same effect was not studied. However, the rational for improved communication among the health care team has been linked to reduced length of stay and hospital costs.

Clinical Implications

Having well-planned and consistent communication is essential for determining seriously ill patients' wishes for care. Using a physician-CNS communication team affected end-of-life resource utilization in this study. Priority must be given to discussing values and plans of care with families and patients as diligently as communicating the technical aspects of patient care.

Family Presence

7. **Wagner J. Lived experience of critically ill patients' family members during cardiopulmonary resuscitation.** *Am J Crit Care.* **2004;13: 416-420.**

Study Sample

Six family members whose loved ones survived cardiopulmonary resuscitation consented to an audiotaped interview.

Comparison Studied

This study described the experiences, thoughts, and perceptions of family members of critically ill patients during cardiopulmonary resuscitation (CPR) in the intensive care unit.

Study Procedures

This study was done in the coronary care unit in a 700-bed urban community hospital in northeastern Ohio. Family members who were near the patient when cardiac arrest occurred were interviewed within 24 hours of the resuscitation. During the interview, family members were asked to describe their experiences during the resuscitation. Interviews were transcribed and were analyzed for relevant themes.

Key Results

One major theme emerged: Should we go or should we stay? Which consists of 3 phases: pre-jives (a premonition that something is amiss), here and now, and breaking the rules. Additionally, two subthemes emerged: What is going on? and You do your job. A model, the Family's Experience with Cardiopulmonary Resuscitation, was developed to reflect the research findings.

Study Strengths and Weaknesses

Only family members of successful resuscitation were asked to participate in this study. Both successful and unsuccessful resuscitation attempts become equally important in determining policy and procedure related to family presence. Finding potential subjects limited the sample size.

Clinical Implications

Family members' informational and proximity needs are often ignored during times of crisis as efforts are focused on the patient. Addressing these needs through appropriate interventions, such as family presence, should be implemented and evaluated.

OTHER REFERENCES

General Overview

1. Beach EK, Maloney BH, Plocica AR, et al. The spouse: a factor in recovery after acute myocardial infarction. *Heart Lung.* 1992;21:30-38.
2. Benning CR, Smith A. Psychosocial needs of family members of liver transplant patients. *Clin Nurse Spec.* 1994;8:280-288.
3. Bergbom I, Svensson C, Berggren E, Kamsula M. Patients' and relatives' opinions and feelings about diaries kept by nurses in an intensive care unit: pilot study. *Intensive Crit Care Nurs.* 1999;15:185-191.
4. Bernstein LP. Family-centered care of the critically ill neurological patient. *Crit Care Nurs Clin North Am.* 1990;2:41-50.
5. Bond AE, Draeger CR, Mandleco B, Donnelly M. Needs of family members of patients with severe traumatic brain injury: implications for evidence-based practice. *Crit Care Nurs.* 2003;23:63-72.
6. Chelsa CA. Reconciling technological and family care in critical care nursing. *J Nurs Sch.* 1996;28:199-204.
7. Collopy KS. Advanced practice nurses guiding families through systems. *Crit Care Nurse.* 1999;19: 80-85.
8. Covinsky KE, Goldman L, Cook EF, et al. The impact of serious illness on patients' families. *JAMA.* 1994; 272:1839-1844.
9. Coutu-Wakulczyk G, Chartier L. French validation of the Critical Care Family Needs Inventory. *Heart Lung.* 1990;19:192-196.
10. Dracup K. Are critical care units hazardous to health? *Appl Nurs Res.* 1988;1:14-21.
11. Dracup K. Beyond the patient: caring for families. *Commun Nurs Res.* 2002;35:53-61.
12. Dunkel J, Eisendrath S. Families in ICU: their effect on staff. *Heart Lung.* 1983;12:258-261.
13. Frederickson K. Anxiety transmission in the patient with myocardial infarction. *Heart Lung.* 1989;18: 617-622.
14. Halm MA. Support and reassurance needs: strategies for practice. *Crit Care Nurs Clin North Am.* 1992;4: 633-643.
15. Henneman E, Cardin S. Family-centered critical care: a practical approach to making it happen. *Crit Care Nurse.* 2002;22:12-19.
16. Hickey M. What are the needs of families of critically ill patients? A review of the literature since 1976. *Heart Lung.* 1990;19:401-415.
17. Holden J, Harrison L, Johnson M. Families, nurse and intensive care patients: a review of the literature. *J Clin Nurs.* 2002;11:140-148.
18. Hupcey JE. Establishing the nurse-family relationship in the intensive care unit. *West J Nurs Res.* 1998;20: 180-184.
19. Hupcey J, Penrod J. Going it alone: the experiences of spouses of critically ill patients. *Dimens Crit Care Nurs.* 2000;19:44-49.
20. Jurkovich GJ, Pierce B, Pananen L, et al. Giving bad news: the family perspective. *J Trauma.* 2000;48: 865-870.
21. Kaye J, Heald G, Polivka D. Spirituality among family members of critically ill adults [abstract]. *Am J Crit Care.* 1996;5:242.
22. Lange MP. Family stress in the intensive care unit. *Crit Care Med.* 2001;29:2025-2026.
23. Leavitt MB. Transition to illness: the family in the hospital. In: Gilliss CL, Highley BL, Roberts BM, Martinson IM, eds. *Toward a Science of Family Nursing.* Menlo Park, Calif: Addison-Wesley; 1989:262-283.
24. Leske JS. Internal psychometric properties of the Critical Care Family Needs Inventory. *Heart Lung.* 1991; 20:236-244.
25. Leske JS. The impact of critical injury as described by a spouse: a retrospective case study. *Clin Nurs Res.* 1992;1:385-401.
26. Leske JS. Overview of family needs after critical illness: from assessment to intervention. *AACN Clin Issues Crit Care Nurs.* 1991;2:220-226.
27. Lopez-Fagin L. Critical Care Family Needs Inven-

tory: a cognitive research utilization approach. *Crit Care Nurs*. 1995;15:21-26.

28. Levine C, Zuckerman C. Hands on/hands off: why healthcare professionals depend on families but keep them at arm's length. *J Law Med Ethics*. 2000;28:5-18.

29. Marsden C. Family-centered critical care: an option or obligation? *Am J Crit Care*. 1992;1:115-117.

30. McQuay JE. Support of families who had a loved one suffer a sudden injury, illness, or death. *Crit Care Nurs Clin North Am*. 1995;7:541-547.

31. Miller P, Wikoff R, McMahon M, Garrett MJ, Ringel K. Marital functioning after cardiac surgery. *Heart Lung*. 1990;19:55-61.

32. Moser DK. Social support and cardiac recovery. *J Cardiovasc Nurs*. 1994;9:27-36.

33. Patterson JM. Promoting resilience in families experiencing stress. *Pediatr Clin North Am*. 1995;42:47-63.

34. Rankin SH, Monahan P. Great expectations: perceived social support in couples experiencing cardiac surgery. *Fam Relations*. 1991;40:297-302.

35. Ross CE, Mirowsky P, Goldsteen K. The impact of the family on health: the decade in review. *J Marriage Fam*. 1990;52:1059-1078.

36. Rutledge DN, Donaldson NE, Pravikoff DS. Caring for families of patients in acute or chronic health care settings: part I-principles. *Online J Clin Innov*. 2000;3(2):1-26.

37. Rutledge DN, Donaldson NE, Pravikoff DS. Caring for families of patients in acute or chronic health care settings: part II-interventions. *Online J Clin Innov*. 2000;3(3):1-52.

38. Simpson T. The family as a source of support for the critically ill adult. *AACN Clin Issues Crit Care Nurs*. 1991;2:229-235.

39. Schlump-Urquhart SR. Families experiencing a traumatic accident: implications and nursing management. *AACN Clin Issues Crit Care Nurs*. 1990;1:522-534.

40. Shelby J, Sullivan J, Groussman M, Gray R, Saffle J. Severe burn injury: effects on psychologic and immunologic function in noninjured close relatives. *J Burn Care Rehabil*. 1992;13:58-63.

41. Solursh DS. The family of the trauma victim. *Nurs Clin North Am*. 1990;25:155-162.

42. Swigart V, Lidz C, Butterworth V, Arnold R. Letting go: family willingness to forgo life support. *Heart Lung*. 1996;25:483-494.

43. Titler MG, Cohen MZ, Craft MJ. Impact of adult critical care hospitalization: perceptions of patients, spouses, children, and nurses. *Heart Lung*. 1991;20:174-182.

44. Tracey MF, Ceronsky C. Creating a collaborative environment to care for complex patients and families. *AACN Clin Issues Crit Care*. 2001;12:383-400.

45. Tracey J, Fowler S, Magarelli K. Hope and anxiety of individuals family members of critically ill adults. *Appl Nurs Res*. 1999;12:121-127.

46. Van Horn E, Tesh A. The effect of critical care hospitalization on family members: stress and responses. *Dimens Crit Care Nurs*. 2000;19:40-49.

47. Vassar EK, Grogan JM. The beginnings. *Crit Care Nurs Clin North Am*. 1995;7:511-515.

48. Washington G. Families in crisis. *Nurs Manage*. 2001;32:28-33.

49. Washington GT. Family advocates: caring for families in crisis. *Dimens Crit Care Nurs*. 2001;20:36-40.

Family Assessment

50. Artinian NT. Bypass surgery: families' perceptions. *Appl Nurs Res*. 1988;1:43-44.

51. Azoulay E, Pochard F. Meeting the needs of intensive care unit patients' family members: beyond satisfaction. *Crit Care Med*. 2002;30:2171.

52. Azoulay E, Pochard F, Chevert S, et al. Meeting the needs of intensive care unit patient families: a multicenter study. *Am J Respir Crit Care Med*. 2001;163:135-139.

53. Bijttebier P, Vanoost S, Delva D, et al. Needs of relatives of critical care patients: perceptions of relatives, physicians, and nurses. *Intensive Care Med*. 2000;24:160-165.

54. Bouman CC. Identifying priority concerns of families of ICU patients. *Dimens Crit Care Nurs*. 1984;3:313-319.

55. Callahan HE. Families dealing with advanced heart failure. *Crit Care Nurs Q*. 2003;26:230-243.

56. Chartier L, Coutu-Wakulczyk G. Families in ICU: their needs and anxiety level. *Intensive Care Nurs*. 1989;5:11-18.

57. Con AH, Linden W, Thompson J, et al. The psychology of men and women recovering from coronary artery bypass surgery. *J Cardiopulmonary Rehabil*. 1999;19:152-161.

58. Coulter MA. The needs of family members of patients in intensive care. *Intensive Care Nurs*. 1989;5:4-10.

59. Daley L. The perceived immediate needs of families with relatives in the intensive care setting. *Heart Lung*. 1984;13:231-237.

60. Dhooper S. Identifying and mobilizing social supports for the cardiac patient's family. *J Cardiovasc Nurs*. 1990;5:65-73.

61. Dockter B, Block D, Hovell M, et al. Families and intensive care nurses: comparison of perceptions. *Patient Educ Counseling*. 1988;12:29-36.

62. Elizur Y, Hirsch E. Psychosocial adjustment and mental health two months after coronary artery bypass surgery: a multisystemic analysis of patients' resources. *J Beh Med*. 1999;22:157-177.

63. Engli M, Kirsivali-Farmer K. Needs of family mem-

bers of critically ill patients with and without acute brain injury. *J Neurosci Nurs.* 1993;25:78-85.

64. Forrester DA. Murphy PA, Price DM, Monaghan JF. Critical care family needs: nurse-family member confederate pairs. *Heart Lung.* 1990;19:655-661.

65. Foss KR, Tenholder MF. Expectations and needs of persons with family members in an intensive care unit as opposed to a general ward. *South Med J.* 1993;86:380-384.

66. Freichels TA. Needs of family members of patients in the intensive care unit over time. *Crit Care Nurs Q.* 1991;14:16-29.

67. Friedman MM. Social support sources among older women with heart failure: continuity versus loss over time. *Res Nurse Health.* 1997;20:319-327.

68. Hammond F. Considering the needs of families in the critical care environment. *Aust Crit Care.* 2002;15:42-43.

69. Hardicre J. Nurses' experiences of caring for the relatives of patient in ICU. *Nurs Times.* 1999;99:34-37.

70. Hardicre J. Meeting the needs of families of patients in intensive care units. *Nurs Times.* 2003;99:26-27.

71. Hickey M, Lewandowski L. Critical care nurses' role with families: a descriptive study. *Heart Lung.* 1988;17:670-676.

72. Holahan CJ, Moos RH, Holahan CK, Brennan PL. Social context, coping strategies, and depressive symptoms: an expanded model with cardiac patients. *J Pers Soc Psychol.* 1997;72:918-928.

73. Hunsucker SC, Frank DI, Flannery J. Meeting the needs of rural families during critical illness: the APN's role. *Dimens Crit Care Nurs.* 1999;18:24-32.

74. Hupcey JE. The meaning of social support for the critically ill patient. *Intensive Crit Care Nurs.* 2001;17:206-212.

75. Jamerson PA, Scheilbmeir M, Bott MJ, Crighton F, Hinton RH, Cobb AK. The experiences of families with a relative in the intensive care unit. *Heart Lung.* 1996;25:467-474.

76. Jillings CR. Psychosocial needs of the patient and family. *Crit Care Nurs Clin North Am.* 1990;2:325-330.

77. Johansson I, Hildingh C, Fridlund B. Coping strategies when an adult next-of-kin/close friend is in critical care: a grounded theory analysis. *Intensive Crit Care Nurs.* 2002;18:96-108.

78. Johnson D, Wilson M, Cavanaugh B, et al. Measuring the ability to meet family needs in an intensive care unit. *Crit Care Med.* 1998;26:266-271.

79. Johnson BP. One family's experience with head injury: a phenomenological study. *J Neurosci Nurs.* 1995;27:113-118.

80. Kleinpell RM, Powers MJ. Needs of family members of intensive care unit patients. *Appl Nurs Res.* 1992;5:2-8.

81. Koller PA. Family needs and coping strategies during illness crisis. *AACN Clin Issues Crit Care Nurs.* 1991;2:338-344.

82. Kosco M, Warren N. Critical care nurses' perceptions of family needs met. *Crit Care Nurs Q.* 2000;23:60-72.

83. Lee I, Chien W, Mackenzie A. Needs of families with a relative in a critical care unit in Hong Kong. *J Clin Nurs.* 2000;9:46-54.

84. Leske JS. Needs of relatives of critically ill patients: a follow-up. *Heart Lung.* 1986;15:189-193.

85. Leung K, Chien W, Mackenzie A. Needs of Chinese families of critically ill patients. *West J Nurs Res.* 2000;22:826-840.

86. Lovejoy NC. Roles played by hospital visitors. *Heart Lung.* 1987;16:573-575.

87. Lynn-McHale DJ, Smith A. Comprehensive assessment of families of the critically ill. *AACN Clin Issues Crit Care Nurs.* 1991;2:195-209.

88. Mahoney J. An ethnographic approach to understanding the illness experience of patients with congestive heart failure. *Heart Lung.* 2001;30:429-435.

89. Marsden C, Dracup K. Different perspectives: the effect of heart disease on patients and spouses. *AACN Clin Issues Crit Care Nurs.* 1991;2:285-292.

90. Martensson J, Dracup K. Fridlund B. Decisive situations influencing spouse's support of patients with heart failure: a critical incident technique analysis. *Heart Lung.* 2001;30:341-350.

91. Mathis M. Personal needs of family members of critically ill patients with and without brain injury. *J Neurosurg Nurs.* 1984;16:36-44.

92. McGauney J. Understanding the information needs of patients and their relatives in intensive care units. *Intensive Crit Care Nurs.* 1994;10:186-194.

93. Mendonca D, Warren N. Perceived and unmet needs of critical care family members. *Crit Care Nurs Q.* 1998;21:58-67.

94. Mirr MP. Factors affecting decisions made by family members of patients with severe head injury. *Heart Lung.* 1991;20:229-235.

95. Molter NC. Needs of relatives of critically ill patients: a descriptive study. *Heart Lung.* 1979;8:332-339.

96. Murphy PA, Forrester A, Price DM, Monaghan JF. Empathy of intensive care nurses and critical care family needs assessment. *Heart Lung.* 1992;21:25-30.

97. Neabel B, Bourbonnais F, Dunning J. Family assessment tools: a review of the literature from 1978-1997. *Heart Lung.* 2000;29:196-209.

98. Nolan MT, Cupples SA, Brown MM, Pierce L, Lepley D, Ohler L. Perceived stress and coping strategies among families of cardiac transplant candidates during the organ waiting period. *Heart Lung.* 1991;21:540-547.

99. Norheim C. Family needs of patients having coronary

artery bypass graft surgery during the intraoperative period. *Heart Lung.* 1989;18:622-626.

100. Norris LO, Grove SK. Investigation of selected needs of family members of critically ill patients. *Heart Lung.* 1986;15:194-199.

101. Nyamathi A, Jacoby A, Constancia P, Ruvevich S. Coping and adjustment of spouses of critically ill patients with cardiac disease. *Heart Lung.* 1992;21:160-166.

102. O'Farrell P, Murray J, Hotz S. Psychological distress among spouses of patients undergoing cardiac rehabilitation. *Heart Lung.* 2000;29:97-104.

103. O'Malley P, Favaloro R, Anderson P, et al. Critical care nurse perceptions of family needs. *Heart Lung.* 1991;20:189-201.

104. Paavilainen E, Seppanen S, Kurki P. Family involvement in perioperative nursing of adult patients undergoing emergency surgery. *J Clin Nurs.* 2001;10:230-237.

105. Pelletier ML. The organ donor family members' perception of stressful situations during the organ donation experience. *J Adv Nurs.* 1992;17:90-97.

106. Perez L, Alexander D, Wise L. Interfacility transport of patients admitted to the ICU: perceived needs of family members. *Air Med J.* 2003;22:44-48.

107. Price AM. Intensive care nurses' experiences of assessing and dealing with patients' psychological needs. *Nurs Crit Care.* 2004;9:134-142.

108. Redley B. LeVasseur S, Peters G, Bethune E. Families' needs in emergency departments: instrument development. *J Adv Nurs.* 2003;43:606-615.

109. Redley B, Beanland C. Revising the Critical Care Family Needs Inventory for the emergency department. *J Adv Nurs.* 2003;45:95-104.

110. Redley B, Beanland C, Botti M. Accompanying critically ill relatives in emergency departments. *J Adv Nurs.* 2003;44:88-98.

111. Robb Y. Family nursing in intensive care, part two: the needs of a family with a member in intensive care. *Intensive Crit Care Nurs.* 1998:14:203-207.

112. Ross E, Graydon J. The impact of the wife on caring for a physically ill spouse. *J Women Aging.* 1997;9:23-35.

113. Rogers CD. Needs of relatives of cardiac surgery patients during the critical care phase. *Focus Crit Care.* 1983;10:50-55.

114. Rukholm E, Bailey P, Coutu-Wakulczyk G. Family needs and anxiety in ICU: cultural differences in Northeastern Ontario. *Can J Nurs Res.* 1991;23(3):67-81.

115. Rukholm E, Bailey P, Coutu-Wakulczyk G, Bailey WB. Needs and anxiety levels in relatives of intensive care unit patients. *J Adv Nurs.* 1991;16:920-928.

116. Simpson T. Needs and concerns of families of critically ill adults. *Focus Crit Care.* 1989;16:388-397.

117. Spatt L, Ganas E, Hying S, et al. Informational needs of families of intensive care patients. *Qual Rev Bull.* 1986;12:16-21.

118. Stewart M, Davidson K, Meade D, et al. Myocardial infarction: survivors' and spouses' stress, coping and support. *J Adv Nurs.* 2000;31:1351-1360.

119. Tin M, French P, Leung K. The needs of the family of critically ill neurosurgical patients: a comparison of nurses' and family members' perceptions. *J Neurosci Nurs.* 1999;31:348-256.

120. Walters AJ. A hermeneutic study of the experiences of relatives of critically ill patients. *J Adv Nurs.* 1995;22:998-1005.

121. Warren NA. Perceived needs of the family members in the critical care waiting room. *Crit Care Nurs Q.* 1993;16:56-63.

122. Wilkinson P. A qualitative study to establish the self-perceived needs of family members in a general intensive care unit. *Intensive Crit Care Nurs.* 1995;11:77-86.

Family Interventions

123. Azoulay E, Pochard F, Chevet S, et al. Family participation in care to the critically ill: opinions of families and staff. *Intensive Care Med.* 2003;29:1498-1504.

124. Azoulay E, Pouchard F, Chevet 5, et al. Impact of a family information leaflet on effectiveness of information provided to family members of intensive care unit patients: a multicenter, prospective, randomized, controlled trial. *Am J Respir Crit Care Med.* 2002;165:438-442.

125. Bokinskie JC. Family conferences: a method to diminish transfer anxiety. *J Neurosci Nurs.* 1992;24:129-133.

126. Chavez W, Faber L. Effect of an education-orientation program on family members who visit their significant other in the intensive care unit. *Heart Lung.* 1987;16:92-99.

127. Clark P, Dunbar S. Family partnership intervention: a guide for a family approach to care of patients with heart failure. *AACN Clin Issues.* 2003;14:467-476.

128. Cray L. A collaborative project: initiating a family intervention program in a medical intensive care unit. *Focus Crit Care.* 1989;16:212-218.

129. Daley K, Kleinpell RM, Lawinger S, Casey G. The effect of two nursing interventions on families of ICU patients. *Clin Nurs Res.* 1994;3:414-422.

130. Day LJ, Stannard D. Developing trust and connection with patients and their families. *Crit Care Nurse.* 1999;19:66-70.

131. Driscoll A. Managing post-discharge care at home: an analysis of patients' and their carers' perception of information received during their hospital stay. *J Adv Nurs.* 2000;31:1165-1173.

132. Dusseldorph E, van Eldereran T, Maes S, et al. A

meta-analysis of psychoeducational programs for coronary disease patients. *Health Psychol.* 1999;18: 506-519.

133. Eichhorn DJ, Meyers TA, Guzzetta CE. Family presence during resuscitation: it is time to open the door. *Capsules Comments Crit Care Nurs.* 1995;3(1):8-13.

134. Elliot J, Smith DR. Meeting family needs following severe head injury: a multidisciplinary approach. *J Neurosurg Nurs.* 1985;17:111-113.

135. Furukawa MM. Meeting the needs of the dying patient's family. *Crit Care Nurse.* 1996;16(1):51-57.

136. Gardner D, Stewart N. Staff involvement with families of patients in critical care units. *Heart Lung.* 1978;7:105-110.

137. Gavaghan SR, Carroll DL. Families and critically ill patients and the effects of nursing interventions. *Dimens Crit Care.*2002;21:64-71.

138. Gilliss CL, Neuhaus JM, Hauck WW. Improved family functioning after cardiac surgery: a randomized trial. *Heart Lung.* 1990;19:648-654.

139. Glennon TP, Smith BS. Questions asked by patients and their support groups during family conferences on inpatient rehabilitation units. *Arch Phys Med Rehabil.* 1990;71:600-702.

140. Goodell TT, Hanson SM. Nurse-family interaction in adult critical care: a Bowen family systems perspective. *J Family Nurs.* 1999;5:72-91.

141. Halm MA. Effects of support groups on anxiety of family members during critical illness. *Heart Lung.* 1990;19:62-71.

142. Halm MA. Strategies for developing a family support group. *Focus Crit Care.* 1991;18:444-459.

143. Halm MA, Titler MG. Appropriateness of critical care visitation: perceptions of patients, families, nurses, and physicians. *J Nurs Qual Assur.* 1990;5:25-37.

144. Hartford K, Wong C. What does the literature report about post-discharge telephone interventions by nurses for coronary artery bypass graft surgery and their partners? *Can J Cardiovasc Nurs.* 2000;11:27-35.

145. Hodovanic BH, Reardon D, Reese W, Hedges B. Family crisis intervention program in the medical intensive care unit. *Heart Lung.* 1984;13:243-249.

146. Jansen M, Schmitt NA. Family-focused interventions. *Crit Care Nurs Clin N Am.* 2003;15:347-354.

147. Kanervisto M, Paavilainen E, Astedt-Kurki P. Impact of chronic obstructive pulmonary disease on family functioning. *Heart Lung.* 2003;32:360-367.

148. Lantz I, Severinsson E. The influence of focus group-orientated supervision on intensive care nurses' reflections on family members' needs. *Intensive Crit Care Nurs.* 2001;17:128-137.

149. Ledbetter-Stone M. Family intervention strategies when dealing with futility of treatment issues: a case study. *Crit Care Nurs Q.* 1999;22:45-50.

150. Leith BA. Transfer anxiety in critical care patients and their family members. *Crit Care Nurs.* 1998;18:24-32.

151. Lenz ER, Perkins S. Coronary artery bypass graft surgery patients and their family member caregivers: outcomes of a family-focused staged psychoeducational intervention. *Appl Nurs Res.* 2000;13:142-150.

152. Leske JS. Family member interventions: research challenges. *Heart Lung.* 1991;20:391-393.

153. Leske JS. Treatment for family members in crisis after critical injury. *AACN Clin Issues Crit Care Nurs.* 1998;9:129-139.

154. Leske JS, Heidrich SM. Interventions for aged family members. *Crit Care Nurs Clin North Am.* 1996;8:91-102.

155. Levine C, Zuckerman C. The trouble with families: toward an ethic of accommodation. *Ann Intern Med.* 1999;130:148-152.

156. Macnab AJ, Emerton-Downey J, Phillips N, Susak LE. Purpose of family photographs displayed in the pediatric intensive care unit. *Heart Lung.* 1997;26:68-75.

157. McGaughey J, Harrison S. Developing an information booklet to meet the needs of intensive care patients and relatives. *Intensive Crit Care Nurs.* 1994;10:271-277.

158. McQuay JE, Schwartz R, Goldblatt PC, Giangrasso VM. 'Death-telling' research project. *Crit Care Nurs Clin North Am.* 1995;7:549-555.

159. Menkhaus S, Turner N, Gueldner S, Michele Y. Effectiveness of the family beeper program (FBP) in the critical care unit [abstract]. *Am J Crit Care.* 1996; 5:236.

160. Moseley MJ, Jones AM. Contracting for visitation with families. *Dimens Crit Care Nurs.* 1991;10:364-371.

161. Nystrom K, Funk M, Sexton D. Patients' perceptions of the adequacy and importance of preoperative instruction before coronary artery bypass graft surgery [abstract]. *Am J Crit Care.* 1996;5:237

162. O'Keefe B, Gilliss CL. Family care in the coronary care unit: an analysis of clinical nurse specialist intervention. *Heart Lung.* 1988;17:191-198.

163. Olson D. Paging the family: using technology to enhance communication. *Crit Care Nurse.* 1997;17(1): 39-41.

164. Palazzo MO. Teaching in crisis: patient and family education in critical care. *Crit Care Nurs Clin North Am.* 2001;13:83-92.

165. Parent N, Fortin F. A randomized, controlled trial of vicarious experience through peer support for male first-time cardiac surgery patients: impact on anxiety, self-efficacy expectation, and self-reported anxiety. *Heart Lung.* 2000;29:389-400.

166. Paul F, Hendrey C, Cabrelli L. Meeting patient and relatives' information needs upon transfer from an intensive care unit: the development and evaluation

of an information booklet. *J Clin Nurs.* 2004;13:396-405.

167. Petterson M. Visual tools for families: a picture is worth a thousand words. *Crit Care Nurs.* 2000:13:83-92.

168. Robinson CA, Thorne S. Strengthening family 'interference.' *J Adv Nurs.* 1984;9:597-602.

169. Roebuck A. Telephone support in the early post-discharge period following elective cardiac surgery: does it reduce anxiety and depression levels? *Intens Crit Care Nurs.* 1999;15:142-146.

170. Sagehorn K, Russell C, Ganong L. Implementation of a patient-family pathway: effects on patients and families. *Clin Nurse Spec.* 1999;13:119-122.

171. Simpson T, Shaver J. Cardiovascular responses to family visits in coronary care unit patients. *Heart Lung.* 1990;19:344-351.

172. Snyder M, Brandt CL, Tseng Y. Use of presence in the critical care unit. *AACN Clin Issues.* 2000;11:27-33.

173. Stewart M, Davidson K, Meade D, et al. Group support for couples coping with a cardiac condition. *J Adv Nurs.* 2001;33:190-199.

174. Thompson DR. Effect of in-hospital counseling on knowledge in myocardial infarction patients and spouses. *Patient Educ Counseling.* 1991;18:171-177.

175. Thompson DR, Meddis R. Wives' responses to counseling early after myocardial infarction. *J Psychosom Res.* 1990;34:249-256.

176. Van Horn E, Fleury J, Moore S. Family interventions during the trajectory of recovery from cardiac event: an integrative literature review. *Heart Lung.* 2002;31:186-198.

177. Ward CR, Constancia P, Kern L. Nursing interventions for families of cardiac surgery patients. *J Cardiovasc Nurs.* 1990;5:34-42.

178. CM. Professional nursing support for culturally diverse family members of critically ill adults. *Res Nurse Health.* 1999;2:107-117.

179. Wesson JS. Meeting the informational, psychosocial and emotional needs of each and family. *Intensive Crit Care Nurs.* 1997;13:111-118.

180. Westphal CG. Storyboards: a teaching strategy for families in critical care. *Dimens Crit Care Nurs.* 1995;14:214-221.

181. Ziemann KM, Dracup K. Patient-nurse contracts in critical care: a controlled trial. *Prog Cardiovasc Nurs.* 1990;5(3):98-103.

Evaluation of Family Satisfaction

182. Artinian NT. Spouses' perceptions of readiness for discharge after cardiac surgery. *Appl Nurs Res.* 1993;6:80-88.

183. Berenholz S, Dorman T, Ngo K, et al. Qualitative review of intensive care unit quality indicators. *J Crit Care.* 2002;17:1-15.

184. Chesla CA, Stannard D. Breakdowns in the nursing care of families in the ICU. *Am J Crit Care.* 1997;6:64-71.

185. Greeneich DS, Long CO. Using a model to assess family satisfaction. *Dimens Crit Care Nurs.* 1993;12:272-278.

186. Heyland D, Tranmer J. Measuring family satisfaction with care in the intensive care unit: the development of a questionnaire and preliminary results. *J Crit Care.* 2001;16:142-149.

187. Hilbert GA. Family satisfaction and affect of men and their wives after myocardial infarction. *Heart Lung.* 1993;22:200-205.

188. Hupcey JE. The need to know: experiences of critically ill patient. Am J Crit Care. 2000;9:192-198.

189. Krumberger JM. Linking critical care family research to quality assurance. *AACN Clin Issues Crit Care Nurs.* 1991;2:321-328.

190. Long CO, Greeneich DS. Family satisfaction techniques: meeting family expectations. *Dimens Crit Care Nurs.* 1994;13:104-111.

191. Lynn-McHale DJ, Bellinger A. Need satisfaction levels of family members of critical care patients and accuracy of nurses' perceptions. *Heart Lung.* 1988;17:447-453.

192. Malacrida R, Bettelini CM, Degrate A, et al. Reasons for dissatisfaction: a survey of relatives of intensive care unit patients who died. Crit Care Med. 1998;26:1187-1193.

193. Martensson J, Dracup K, Fridlund B. Decisive situations influencing spouses' support of patients with heart failure: a critical incident technique analysis. *Heart Lung.* 2001;30:341-350.

194. Wasser T, Matchett S. Final version of the Critical Care Family Satisfaction Survey questionnaire. *Crit Care Med.* 2001;29:1654-1655.

Evaluation of Family Outcomes

195. Azoulay E, Chevret S, Leleu G, et al. Half the families of intensive care unit patients experience inadequate communication with physicians. *Crit Care Med.* 2000;28:3044-3049.

196. Bull MJ, Hansen HE, Gross CR. Differences in family caregiving outcomes by the level of involvement in discharge planning. *App Nurs Res.* 2000;13:76-82.

197. Chaboyer W, Grace J. Following the path of ICU survivors: a quality-improvement activity. *Nurs Crit Care.* 2003;8:149-155.

198. Davies N. Patients' and carers' perceptions of factors influencing recovery after cardiac surgery. *J Adv Nurs.* 2000;32:318-326.

199. Dejong W, Franz H, Wolfe S, et al. Requesting organ

donation: an interview study of donor and nondonor families. *Am J Crit Care*. 1998;7:13-23.

200. Fink SV. The influence of family resources and family demands on the strains and well-being of caregiving families. *Nurs Res*. 1995;44139-146.

201. Fiscella K, Campbell TL. Association of perceived family criticism with health behaviors. *J Family Practice*. 199;48:128-134.

202. Giuliano KK, Giuliano AJ, Bloniasz E, et al. A quality-improvement approach to meeting the needs of critically ill patients and their families. *Dimens Crit Care Nurs*. 2000;19:30-34.

203. Grossman M. Received support and psychological adjustment in critically injured patients and their family. *J Neurosci Nurs*. 1995;27:11-23.

204. Hall-Smith J, Ball C, Coakley J. Follow-up services and the development of a clinical nurse specialist in critical care. *Intensive Crit Care Nurs*. 1997;13:243-248.

205. Halm M, Gagner S, Goering M, et al. Interdisciplinary rounds: impact on patients, families, and staff. *Clin Nurse Spec*. 2003;17:133-142.

206. Hupcey JE. Feeling safe: the psychosocial needs of ICU patients. *J Nurs Sch*. 2000;32:361-367.

207. Johnson P, Chaboyer W, Foster M, et al. Caregivers of ICU patients discharged home: what burden do they face? *Intensive Crit Care Nurs*. 2001;17:219-227.

208. Jones C, Skirrow P, Griffiths RD, et al. Post-traumatic stress disorder-related symptoms in relatives of patients following intensive care. *Intensive Care Med*. 2004;30:456-460.

209. Leske JS. Family stresses, strengths, and outcomes after critical injury. *Crit Care Nurs Clin North Am*. 2000;12:237-244.

210. Leske JS, Jiricka MK. Impact of family demands and family strengths and capabilities on family well-being and adaptation after critical injury. *Am J Crit Care*. 1998;7:383-392.

211. Leith B. Patients' and family members' perceptions of transfer from intensive care. *Heart Lung*. 1999;28:210-218.

212. Mitchell M, Courtney M, Coyer F. Understanding uncertainty and minimizing families' anxiety at the time of transfer from intensive care. *Nurs Health Sci*. 2003;5:207-217.

213. Rantanen A, Kaunonen M, Astedt-Kurki P, et al. Coronary artery bypass grafting: social support for patients and their significant others. *J Clin Nurs*. 2004;13:158-166.

214. Russell S. Continuity of care after discharge from ICU. *Prof Nurs*. 2000;15:497-500.

215. Saunders MM. Family caregivers need support with heart failure patients. *Holist Nurs Pract*. 2003;17:136-142.

216. Strahan E, McCormick J, Uprichard E, et al. Immedi-ate follow-up after ICU discharge: establishment of a service and initial experiences. *Nurs Crit Care*. 2003;8:49-55.

217. Tarkka M, Paavilainen E, Lehti K, et al. In-hospital support for families of heart patients. *J Clin Nurs*. 2002;12:736-743.

218. Twibell RS. Family coping during critical illness. *Dimens Crit Care*. 1998;17:100-112.

End-of-Life Care

219. Abbott K, Sago J, Breen C, et al. Families looking back: one year after discussion of withdrawal or withholding of life-sustaining support. *Crit Care Med*. 2001;29:197-200.

220. Andrew CM. Optimizing the human experience: nursing the families of people who die in intensive care. *Intensive Crit Care Nurs*. 1998;14:59-65.

221. Bradley EH, Cherlin F, McCorkel R, et al. Nurses' use of palliative care practices in the acute care setting. *J Prof Nurs*. 2001;17:14-22.

222. Counsell C, Guin P. Exploring family needs during withdrawal of life support in critically ill patients. *Crit Care Nurs Clin North Am*. 2002;14:187-192.

223. Curtis, JR, Patrick DL, Shannon SE, et al. The family conference as a focus to improve communication about end-of-life care in the intensive care unit: opportunities for improvement. *Crit Care Med*. 2001;29(2 suppl):26-33.

224. Dejong W, Franz H, Wolfe S, et al. Requesting organ donation: an interview study of donor and nondonor families. *Am J Crit Care*. 1998; 7:13-23.

225. Kirchoff KT, Beckstrand R. Critical care nurses' perceptions of obstacles and helpful behaviors in providing end-of-life care to dying patients. *Am J Crit Care*. 2000;9:96-105.

226. Kirchoff K, Spuhler V, Walker L, et al. Intensive care nurses' experiences with end-of-life care. *Am J Crit Care*. 2000;9:36-42.

227. Malacrida R, Bettelini CM, Degrate A, et al. Reasons for dissatisfaction: a survey of relatives of intensive care patients who died. *Crit Care Med*. 1998;26:1187-1193.

228. Pochard F, Azoulay E, Chevret S, et al. Symptoms of anxiety and depression in family members of intensive care unit patients: ethical hypothesis regarding decision-making capacity. *Crit Care Med*. 2001;29:1893-1897.

229. Riley LP, Coolican MB. Needs of families of organ donors: facing death and life. *Crit Care Nurs Q*. 1999;19:53-59.

230. Tastremski CA. Caring for the families of those who die in the critical care unit. *Crit Care Med*. 1998;26:1150-1151.

231. Tilden VP, Tolle SW, Nelson CA, et al. Family decision making in foregoing life extending treatments. *J Family Nurs*. 1999;5:426-442.

232. Warren NA. Critical care family members' satisfaction with bereavement experiences. *Crit Care Nurs Q.* 2002;25:54-60.

Family Presence

233. American Heart Association. Guidelines 2000 for cardiopulmonary resuscitation and emergency cardiovascular care. *Circulation.* 2000;102(suppl 8):1-374.

234. American Heart Association. Ethical aspects of CPR and ECC. *Circulation.* 2000;102:1-12.

237. Bauchner H, Vinci R, Bak S, et al. Parents and procedures: a randomized control trial. *Pediatrics.* 1996;98: 861-886.

238. Barratt F, Wallis DN. Relatives in the resuscitation room: their point of view. *J Accid Emer Med.* 1998; 15:109-123.

239. Belanger MA, Reed S. A rural community hospital's experience with family-witnessed resuscitation. *J Emerg Nurs.* 1997;3:238-239.

240. Boyd R, White S. Does witnessed cardiopulmonary resuscitation alter perceived stress in accident and emergency staff? *J Accid Emerg Med.* 1998;15: 109-110.

241. Boudreaux E, Francis J, Loyacano T. Family presence during invasive procedures and resuscitations in the emergency department: a critical review and suggestions for the future. *Ann Emerg Med.* 2002;40: 193-205.

242. Clark AP, Calvin AO, Meyers TA, et al., Family presence during cardiopulmonary resuscitation and invasive procedures: a research-based intervention. *Crit Care Nurs Clin North Am.* 2001;**13**:569-575.

243. Doyle CJ, Post H, Burney R, et al. Family presence during resuscitation: an option. *Ann Emerg Med.* 1987; 16:673-675.

244. Eckle N, MacLean S. Assessment of family-centered care for pediatric patients in the emergency department. *J Emerg Nurs.* 2001;27:238-245.

245. Eichhorn, DJ, Meyers TA, Mitchell TG, Guzzetta CE. Opening the doors: family presence during resuscitation. *J Cardiovasc Nurs.* 1996;10:59-70.

246. Ellison S. Nurses' attitudes toward family presence during resuscitative efforts and invasive procedures. *J Emerg Nurs.* 2003;29:515-521.

247. Emergency Nurses Association. *Presenting the Option of Family Presence.* 2nd ed. Des Plaines, Ill: The Emergency Nurses Association; 2001.

248. Gulranjani RP. Physical environmental factors affecting patient's stress in the accident and emergency department. *J Accid Emerg Nurs.* 1995;22-27.

249. Guzzetta CE, Mitchell TG. Response to high touch in high tech: the presence of relatives and friends during resuscitative efforts. *Sch Inq Nurs Pract.* 1997;11: 169-173.

250. Hallgrimsdottir, EM. Accident and emergency nurses' perceptions and experiences of caring for families. *J Clin Nurs.* 2000;9:611-619.

251. Hallgrimsdottir EM. Caring for families in A & E departments: Scottish and Icelandic nurses opinions and experiences. *J Accid Emerg Nurs.* 2004;12:114-120.

252. Hanson C, Strawser D. Family presence during cardiopulmonary resuscitation: Foote hospital emergency department's nine-year perspective. *J Emerg Nurs.* 1992;18:104-106.

253. Helmer SD, Shapiro, WM, Dors JM, Karan, BS. Family presence during trauma resuscitation: a survey of AAST and ENA members. *J Trauma Injury Infect Crit Care.* 2000;48:1015-1020.

254. Institute for Family-Centered Care. Family-centered care: questions and answers. *Adv Family-Centered Care.* 1999;5:2-4.

255. McClenathan B, Torrington K, Uyejara C. Family member presence during cardiopulmonary : a survey of US and international critical care professionals. *Chest.* 2002;122:2204-2210.

256. Meyers TA, Eichhorn DJ, Guzzetta CE. Do families want to be present during CPR? A retrospective survey. *J Emerg Nurs.* 1998;24: 400-405.

257. Mitchell M, Lynch M. Should relatives be allowed in the resuscitation room? *J Accid Emerg Med.* 1997;14:366-369.

258. Moorse J, Pooler C. Patient-family-nurse interactions in the trauma-resuscitation room. *Am J Crit Care.* 2002;11:240-249.

259. Moreland P. Family presence during invasive procedures and resuscitation in the emergency department: a review of the literature. *J Emerg Nurs.* In Press.

260. O'Brien M, Creamer K, Hill E, Welham J. Tolerance of family presence during pediatric. Cardiopulmonary resuscitation: a snapshot of military and civilian pediatricians, nurses, and residents. *Pediatr Emerg Care.* 2002;7:51-53.

261. O'Brien J, Fothergill-Bourbonnais F. The experience of trauma resuscitation in the emergency department: themes from seven patients. *J Emerg Nurs.* 2004;30: 216-224.

262. Osuagwu CC. ED codes: keep the family out. *J Emerg Nurs.* 1991;17:363.

263. Peterson M. Family presence protocol can be a powerful healing force. *Crit Care Nurs.* 1999;19:104.

264. Powers KS, Rubenstein JS. Family presence during invasive procedures in the pediatric intensive care unit. *Arch Pediatr Adolesc Med.* 1999; 153:955-958.

265. Redley B, Hood K. Staff attitudes towards family presence during resuscitation. *J Accid Emerg Nurs.* 1997;4:145-151.

266. Redley B, Botti M, Duke M. Family member presence during resuscitation in the emergency department: an Australia perspective. *Emerg Med Australia.* 2004:16: 295-298.

267. Reynolds D. Death as a shared experience. *ED Management.* 1992;14:177-181.

268. Rosenczweig, C. Should relatives witness resuscitation? Ethical issues and practice considerations. *Can Med Assoc J.* 1998;158-617-620.

269. Sacchetti AD, Lichenstein R, Carraccio CA, et al. Family member presence during pediatric emergency department procedures. *Pediatr Emerg Care.* 1996;12:268-271.

270. Sacchetti AD, Guzzetta CE, Harris RH. Family presence during resuscitation attempts: is there science behind the emotion? *Clin Ped Emer Med.* 2003;4:292-296.

271. Timmermans S. High touch in high tech: The presence of relatives and friends during resuscitation efforts. *Sch Inq Nurs Pract.* 1997;11:53-68.

272. Turner P. Establishing a protocol for parental presence in recovery. *Br J Nurs.* 1997;6:794-799.

273. Tye C. Qualified nurses' perceptions of the needs of suddenly bereaved family members in the accident and emergency department. *J Adv Nurs.* 1993;18:948-956.

274. Van der Woning M. Should relatives be invited to witness a resuscitation attempt? *J Accid Emerg Nurs.* 1997;5:215-218.

275. Williams J. Family presence during resuscitation: to see or not to see? *Nurs Clin North Am.* 2002;37:211-220.

276. Carr JM, Clarke P. Development of the concept of family vigilance. *West J Nurs Res.* 1997;19:726-739.

277. Chesla CA, Stannard D. Breakdown in the nursing care of families in the ICU. *Am J Crit Care.* 1997;6:64-71.

278. Walters AJ. The lifeworld of relatives of critically ill patients: a phenomenology hermeneutic study. *Int J Nurs Prac.* 1995;1:18-25.

279. Warren NA. The phenomena of nurses' caring behaviors as perceived by the critical care family. *Crit Care Nurs Q.* 1994;17(3):67-72.

280. Artinian NT. Stress experience of spouses of patients having coronary artery bypass during hospitalization and six weeks after discharge. *Heart Lung.* 1991;20:52-59.

281. Davis-Martin S. Perceived needs of families of long-term critical care patients: a brief report. *Heart Lung.* 1994;23:515-518.

282. Gordon H, Rosenthal G. Impact of marital status on outcomes in hospitalized patients: evidence from an academic medical center. *Arch Intern Med.* 1995;155:2465-2471.

283. Jacono J, Hicks G, Antonioni C, O'Brien K, Rasi M. Comparison of perceived needs of family members between registered nurses and family members of critically ill patients in intensive care and neonatal intensive care units. *Heart Lung.* 1990;19:72-78.

284. Johnson SK, Craft M, Titler M, et al. Perceived changes in adult family members' roles and responsibilities during critical illness. *Image J Nurs Sch.* 1995;27:238-243.

285. Kleiber C, Halm M, Titler M, et al. Emotional responses of family members during a critical care hospitalization. *Am J Crit Care.* 1994;3:70-76.

286. Leavitt MB. Family recovery after vascular surgery. *Heart Lung.* 1990;19:486-490.

287. Leske JS. Comparison rating of need importance after critical illness from family members with varied demographic characteristics. *Crit Care Nurs Clin N Am.* 1992;4:607-613.

288. Pelletier ML. The needs of family members of organ and tissue donors. *Heart Lung.* 1993;3:151-157.

289. Reider JA. Anxiety during critical illness of a family member. *Dimens Crit Care Nurs.* 1994;13:272-279.

290. Servio CD, Kreutzer JS, Gervasio AH. Predicting family needs after brain injury: implications for intervention. *J Head Trauma Rehabil.* 1995;10(2):32-45.

291. Appleyard ME, et al. Nurse-coached intervention for families of patients in critical care units. *Crit Care Nurs.* 2000;20:40-48.

292. Chavez, CW, Faber L. Effect of an education-orientation program on family members who visit their significant other in the intensive care unit. *Heart Lung.* 1987;16:92-99.

293. Field BE, Devich LE, Carlson RW. Impact of a comprehensive supportive care team on management of hopelessly ill patients with multiple organ failure. *Chest.* 1989;96:353-356.

294. Gillis CL, Neuhaus JM, Hauck WW. Improved family functioning after cardiac surgery: a randomized trial. *Heart Lung.* 1990;19:648-654.

295. Halm MA. Effects of support groups on anxiety of family members during critical illness. *Heart Lung.* 1990;19:62-71.

296. Hartford K, Wong C, Zakaria D. Randomized control trial of a telephone intervention by nurses to provide information and support to patients and their family partners after elective coronary artery bypass graft surgery: effects of anxiety. *Heart Lung.* 2002;31:199-206.

297. Henneman EA, McKenzie JB, Dewa CS. An evaluation of interventions for meeting the information needs of families of critically ill patients. *Am J Crit Care.* 1992;3:85-93.

298. Keeling AW, Dennison PD. Nurse-initiated telephone follow-up after acute myocardial infarction: a pilot study. *Heart Lung.* 1995;24:45-49.

299. Medland JJ, Ferrans CE. Effectiveness of a structured communication program for family members of patients in ICU. *Am J Crit Care.* 1998;7:24-29.

300. Raleigh E, Lepczyk M, Rowley C. Significant others benefit from preoperative information. *J Adv Nurs.* 1990;15:941-945.

301. Sabo KA, Kraay C, Rudy E, et al. ICU family support group sessions: family members' perceived benefits. *Appl Nurs Res*. 1989;2:82-89.

302. Topp R, Walsh E, Sanford C. Can providing paging devices relieve waiting room anxiety? *AORN J*. 1998; 67:852-861.

303. Heyland D, Rocker G, Dodek P, et al. Family satisfaction with care in the intensive care unit: results of a multiple center study. *Crit Care Med*. 2002;30:1413-1418.

304. Hupcey JE. Looking out for the patient and ourselves-the process of family integration into the ICU. *J Clin Nurs*. 1999;8:253-262.

305. Leske JS. Comparison of family stresses, strengths, and outcomes after trauma and surgery. *AACN Clin Issues Crit Care Nurs*. 2003;14:33-41.

306. Jacob DA. Family members' experiences with decision making for incompetent patients in the ICU: a qualitative study. *Am J Crit Care*. 1998;7:30-36.

307. Bassler PC. The impact of education on nurses' beliefs regarding family presence in a resuscitation room. *J Nurs Staff Dev*. 1999;15:131-138.

308. Eichorn DJ, Meyers TA, Guzzetta CE, et al. Family presence during invasive procedures and resuscitation: hearing the voice of the patient. *Am J Nurs*. 2000;101:26-33.

309. MacLean S, Guzzetta C, White C, et al. Family presence during cardiopulmonary resuscitation and invasive procedures: practices of critical care and emergency nurses. *Am J Crit Care*. 2003;12:246-257.

310. Meyers TA, Eichorn D, Guzzetta CE. Family presence during invasive procedures and resuscitation: the experience of family members, nurses, and physicians. *Am J Nurs*. 2000;100:32-42.

311. Robinson S, MacKenzie-Ross S, Campbell-Hawson G, et al. Psychological effect of witnessed resuscitation on bereaved relatives. *Lancet*. 1998;352:614-617.

312. Clark AP, Aldridge MD, Guzetta CE, et al. Family presence during cardiopulmonary resuscitation. *Crit Care Nurs Clin N Am*. 2005;17:23-32.

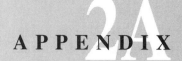
Critical Care Needs Inventory

Please check ( ) how **IMPORTANT** each of the following needs is to you.	Not Important (1)	Slightly Important (2)	Important (3)	Very Important (4)
1. To know the expected outcome	_____	_____	_____	_____
2. To have explanations of the environment before going into the critical care unit for the first time	_____	_____	_____	_____
3. To talk to the doctor every day	_____	_____	_____	_____
4. To have a specific person to call at the hospital when unable to visit	_____	_____	_____	_____
5. To have questions answered honestly	_____	_____	_____	_____
6. To have visiting hours changed for special conditions	_____	_____	_____	_____
7. To talk about feelings about what has happened	_____	_____	_____	_____
8. To have good food available in the hospital	_____	_____	_____	_____
9. To have directions as to what to do at the bedside	_____	_____	_____	_____
10. To visit at any time	_____	_____	_____	_____
11. To know which staff members could give what type of information	_____	_____	_____	_____
12. To have friends nearby for support	_____	_____	_____	_____
13. To know why things were done for the patient	_____	_____	_____	_____

Please check ( ) how **IMPORTANT** each of the following needs is to you.	Not Important (1)	Slightly Important (2)	Important (3)	Very Important (4)
14. To feel there is hope	_____	_____	_____	_____
15. To know about the types of staff members taking care of the patient	_____	_____	_____	_____
16. To know how the patient is being treated medically	_____	_____	_____	_____
17. To be assured that the best care possible is being given to the patient	_____	_____	_____	_____
18. To have a place to be alone while in the hospital	_____	_____	_____	_____
19. To know exactly what is being done for the patient	_____	_____	_____	_____
20. To have comfortable furniture in the waiting room	_____	_____	_____	_____
21. To feel accepted by the hospital staff	_____	_____	_____	_____
22. To have someone to help with financial problems	_____	_____	_____	_____
23. To have a telephone near the waiting room	_____	_____	_____	_____
24. To have a pastor visit	_____	_____	_____	_____
25. To talk about the possibility of the patient's death	_____	_____	_____	_____
26. To have another person with you when visiting the critical care unit	_____	_____	_____	_____
27. To have someone be concerned with your health	_____	_____	_____	_____
28. To be assured it is alright to leave the hospital for awhile	_____	_____	_____	_____
29. To talk to the same nurse every day	_____	_____	_____	_____
30. To feel it is alright to cry	_____	_____	_____	_____
31. To be told about other people that could help with problems	_____	_____	_____	_____
32. To have a bathroom near the waiting room	_____	_____	_____	_____
33. To be alone at any time	_____	_____	_____	_____
34. To be told about someone to help with family problems	_____	_____	_____	_____
35. To have explanations given that are understandable	_____	_____	_____	_____
36. To have visiting hours start on time	_____	_____	_____	_____
37. To be told about chaplain services	_____	_____	_____	_____
38. To help with the patient's physical care	_____	_____	_____	_____

Please check ( ) how **IMPORTANT** each of the following needs is to you.	Not Important (1)	Slightly Important (2)	Important (3)	Very Important (4)
39. To be told about transfer plans while they are being made	_____	_____	_____	_____
40. To be called at home about changes in the patient's condition	_____	_____	_____	_____
41. To receive information about the patient at least once a day	_____	_____	_____	_____
42. To feel that the hospital personnel care about the patient	_____	_____	_____	_____
43. To know specific facts concerning the patient's progress	_____	_____	_____	_____
44. To see the patient frequently	_____	_____	_____	_____
45. To have the waiting room near the patient	_____	_____	_____	_____
46. Other				

Family Visitation and Partnership

Monica A. Redekopp, MN, RN

Jane Stover Leske, RN, PhD

Family Visitation and Partnership

CASE STUDY

It was a crisp Saturday in Fall when the lives of the Ellenger family changed dramatically. Dave and his wife Sandy, with their two little girls Angela, 3, and Terry, 2, were on their way to Sandy's parents' farm when they were hit by a truck as they turned off the busy highway into the driveway. Grandpa was first on the scene and called the local rescue team. Sandy and her children were transported to the local emergency department (ED) of a 500-bed hospital. When Dave, grandpa, and grandma got to the ED they learned that Sandy had been dead on arrival, Angela was in surgery for a depressed skull fracture, and Terry was unconscious with closed head injuries. Sandy's nine siblings were notified of the accident, but not the death, and were requested by their parents not to come to the hospital.

Sandy's sister Mary, who had been her maid of honor, often babysat for the two girls. Sandy was her best friend and mentor. Mary sensed that something was terribly wrong and went to the ED, not knowing that her sister and best friend had died.

The first person Mary met in the ED was a chaplain who asked Mary who she was. When she informed him that she was looking for her sister Sandy, he escorted her to her parents. The rest of the ED encounter was a blur for Mary. She was told that Terry was being transported to the ICU, that Angela was still in surgery, and that Dave was with Sandy. After a long period of confusion and overwhelming grief in the ED, Mary went with her parents to the ICU waiting room. Although Mary wanted to see Terry and Angela, she was politely informed that visiting in the ICU was for immediate family only. After sitting for several hours in vigilance in the ICU waiting room, Mary was persuaded by her parents to return home with the other siblings. Mary's parents

arrived home late that night with the report that Angela and Terry would be fine. Mary was relieved.

Mary awoke the next morning to be told by her father that Angela had died at 5:00 that morning. Mary was sure there was a mistake. She was distraught and angry that she had not stayed to see Angela, and now it was too late.

Mary got dressed and went to the hospital to see Terry. When she was stopped at the door of the ICU and asked if she was immediate family, she lied and said yes. She approached Terry's bedside cautiously, noting that she appeared to be sleeping. The nurse informed her that Terry was still very drowsy from the bump on her head. Mary sat at her bedside, holding her hand for what seemed like a very short time, when the nurse notified her that the 10 minutes of visiting was over. After pleading, with tears in her eyes, to stay just a few more minutes the nurse let her stay. Mary left after another 15 minutes, feeling better now that she had seen Terry and knowing, based on the information the nurse gave her, that Terry would probably recover fully.

Although this true story happened more than 20 years ago, how many critical care units (CCUs) still have restricted visiting? How often do nurses treat family members as visitors and limit interactions between patients and their loved ones? How can nurses promote family-centered interactions in a critical care setting?

GENERAL DESCRIPTION

Visiting continues to be a major issue in critical care practice. During the 1960s, the US Public Health service recommended that visiting in ICUs be restricted to immediate family members for short periods of time, and that a waiting room be provided close to the ICU (Other References: 18). Although family-focused care is a rapidly emerging concept in today's health care system, the systems of critical care are designed for the work of staff and to meet the physiological needs of patients rather than to promote family-centered care. Patients and their families are not usually treated as units, and some nurses believe that family visitors can negatively influence the well-being of the patient (Annotated Bibliography: 3; Other References: 21, 71).

Historically, children have been restricted from visiting in adult CCUs and special care nurseries because it was believed that the visit would be too psychologically stressful or epidemiologically unsafe for the child and the critically ill adult or neonate. Studies suggest, however, that children who are screened for communicable illnesses before visiting are no more likely than adults to spread infection (Other References: 39, 66, 76). Others are concerned about potential psychological stress on the child who visits. They worry that visiting a critically ill adult or sibling may result in extreme behavioral and emotional responses with long-term trauma to the child. Some critical care nurses believe that children should visit so they can obtain direct visual and verbal information about the condition of the critically ill, and allow children to visit despite hospital policy restricting such visits (Other References: 17).

Parental beliefs about hospital visitation by children vary. Some parents withhold information from their children, thinking it might be upsetting. However, children are very curious about their ill family member. They have many questions about the meaning of the illness and the probable outcomes for both patient and family (Other References: 64, 78).

Promoting proximity between the patient and family members is an important component of family-centered care. Family members are defined as adults, children, and family pets. In a landmark study by Leske (Other References: 26, 29), visiting needs are clustered with other selected information needs and are termed *proximity*—the need to have personal contact and to remain near the critically ill person, physically and emotionally. Thus, facilitating visiting between the critically ill patient and family members is a process of instituting change in order for family members to interact with their critically ill loved one.

Adult Critically Ill Patients and Visitation by Adults

Surveys examining visiting policies of various adult ICUs reveal a diversity of visitation practices in which nurses frequently bend the rules (Annotated Bibliography: 6). There is no consensus on the ideal visiting policy. Some experts suggest that family members should not be viewed as visitors but rather incorporated as part of care delivery (Suggested Readings: 8).

Rigid visiting restrictions should be abolished. Research shows that restricted visitation in the adult ICU is based on tradition and actually may be harmful to patients, family members, and family dynamics. Adverse patient responses to visiting, as documented by some investigators, may decrease when visiting is controlled by patients and their

family members. Restricting visiting to short periods and terminating visits prematurely contributes to adverse hemodynamic consequences in critically ill adult patients (Suggested Readings: 17).

Nurses sometimes justify restrictive visiting practices as protecting the patient from adverse physiological consequences, but recent research does not support this assumption. Cardiovascular responses of patients to visitors, compared to nurse-patient or other comparable interactions, are not harmful to the patient (Annotated Bibliography: 5; Other References: 60, 74, 75). Two studies have shown a decline in cardiovascular parameters from visiting by family members (Annotated Bibliography: 5; Other References: 74) while other studies (Other References: 38, 62, 69) have documented that patients' intracranial pressure decreased during patient-family interaction.

Movement to less restricted, individualized visiting practices is recommended. An ideal approach considers patient and family visiting preferences, assesses patient and family needs as part of the history and physical exam (Appendix 3-A), and incorporates needs and preferences into the plan of care. Options to restricted visiting include the following:

- *Flexible visiting*—Families and staff reach a mutual understanding about length and time of visits and who visits. Families are encouraged to be at the bedside, showing sensitivity for patient needs, activity level in the unit, and their own need for positive health (Other References: 42; Suggested Readings: 15, 21).
- *Contract*—A written agreement among family, nurse, and patient regarding time; frequency and length of visits; and number, age, and type of visitors (Appendix 3-B). The contract is periodically reviewed and revised (Other References: 6, 36, 80; Suggested Readings: 7, 10).
- *Patient-controlled visitation*—A device is used to signal when the patient wants (green light) and does not want (red light) visitors. Patients may need help in terminating the visit gracefully. This approach is not for all patients; some patients may want to divert decision making to another person (Annotated Bibliography: 4; Suggested Readings: 5).
- *Structured*—Periodic visitation by 2 people for a longer period (eg, 30-60 minutes) than the traditional 5- to 10-minute visit (Other References: 41; Suggested Readings: 15).
- *Inclusive*—Visiting at any time except at standardized, specified hours agreed on by staff (eg, at shift change) (Other References: 41; Suggested Readings: 11, 15).
- *Open visiting*—No restrictions placed on frequency, time, or length of visits. Number and type of visitors may be restricted (Other References: 27).

Revising unit visiting policies is an important part of facilitating interaction between critically ill patients and family members. However, Kirchhoff and colleagues (Annotated Bibliography: 3) note that administrative policy about visiting does not change the behavior of nurses; changing nurses' beliefs and attitudes about visiting must be done first. A successful transition to more flexible visiting practices depends on the positive beliefs and attitudes of the nursing staff. This is exemplified by the process Osborn and Downer (Suggested Readings: 11) used to change visiting practices in their ICU. Perhaps "policy on visiting in critical care" should be replaced with "practice guidelines for visiting." Institutions could then focus on using practice guidelines to facilitate interactions among critically ill patients and family members rather than basing practice on administrative visiting policies.

To promote interaction among critically ill patients and family members, it is important to consider strategies that prepare family members for visiting, such as preoperative preparation for visits following surgical procedures that are likely to require a critical care stay. Preoperative preparation strategies to consider include tours to the critical care unit (CCU); assessing patient preferences for visiting while in the CCU; and use of videotapes and written materials to describe the critical care setting, what to expect immediately following surgery, and what the visiting practices are in the designated unit. See Appendix 3-C for topics to include in materials designed to orient families to the critical care setting.

Child Visitation in the Adult and Neonatal Intensive Care Unit

When a family member is hospitalized with a critical illness, behavioral and emotional responses vary depending on the role of the ill member and the interaction among other members of the family system (Other References: 78). Studies of the responses of children during a family member's illness suggest there are a wide variety of adverse reactions that might be tempered if children were honestly told what had occurred (Other References: 25, 57, 68).

Qualitative studies of the impact of a critical illness on families revealed that parents shield children from receiving information about the critically ill family member. Despite this shielding, children are able to describe with some accuracy what was happening to their loved one (Other References: 64, 78). It therefore seems logical to assume that children would benefit if they knew what was happening and what to expect when visiting a critically ill family member. This finding led to a series of studies by the Family Intervention Research Team at the University of Iowa in which a structured, Facilitated Child Visitation Intervention (FCVI) was tested with children over the age of 5 years.

Results of two studies suggest the FCVI may limit negative or adverse behavioral and emotional reactions in children visiting in CCUs, and the visit appears to lack harmful effects. The FCVI helps children through a visit of a critically ill adult family member by educating them before the visit and providing additional information and support. One study using the FCVI (Other References: 68) showed that 10 children who received the FCVI when visiting a parent or grandparent in the ICU experienced fewer parent-reported behavioral and emotional changes (eg, getting mad or angry, having trouble concentrating or difficulty sleeping) compared to 10 counterparts who were restricted from visiting. In a second study (unpublished data, 1994) of 64 children visiting parents and grandparents in the ICU, no adverse responses were reported for the 32 children receiving the FCVI. Similar studies are available for siblings visiting in special care nurseries (Other References: 33, 70; Suggested Readings: 13). In addition, knowledge accumulated in previous studies on the importance of preparing children for their own hospitalization parallels what has been found in studies using the FCVI (Other References: 14, 43).

Age-appropriate interventions are beneficial in helping to prepare children for what they might see, feel, and hear (Other References: 33, 56, 68, 70; Suggested Readings: 1, 4, 13). This can be done using photos or graphic illustrations of the unit and computer programs, coloring books and story books, and videotape presentations.

When visitation is an option for children, it is important to make sure the child understands what to expect (Suggested Readings: 4, 13; Other References: 70). Expert opinion and empirically based principles and knowledge are used to implement the FCVI for children who choose to visit a critically ill adult or neonate (Suggested Readings: 4, 6, 13; Other References: 70).

COMPETENCY

Adult Critically Ill Patients and Visitation by Adults

Competencies of staff are crucial to facilitate visiting. Nurses receive little formal education or experiential learning about facilitating interaction between critically ill patients and their loved ones. Of 226 critical care nurses surveyed, more than one third said they did not have the required knowledge and skill to meet the psychosocial and emotional needs of families, more than 75% said it was emotionally exhausting to become involved with families, and nearly 40% believed it was unrealistic for critical care staff to care for the emotional needs of the family (Other References: 21). Nurses may be uncomfortable having family members at the bedside while they are performing patient care (Other References: 81, 83). The nurse's priority is to take care of the patient; family members only add confusion to an already busy unit (Annotated Bibliography: 1, 3; Other References: 81). "Perhaps if families were perceived as being 'helpful' to the nurse, they would be allowed to stay longer than the prescribed visiting hours" (Annotated Bibliography: 3, p. 244). Nurses report the following variables about visiting affect their practice: patients' need for rest, nurses' workload, and perceived benefits for patients. Requests for visiting from patients' families were ranked as least important (Other References: 71). For nurses who view families as an encumbrance, the ideal family is cooperative, quiet, and follows the rules (Annotated Bibliography: 1).

Everyone has the patient's best interest at heart, and nurses carrying for critically ill patients need competencies in facilitating patient and family member interaction. Just as IV drips are individualized and titrated according to patient response, so must be visiting in critical care.

First of all, nurses need both a positive attitude about the importance of family-centered critical care and knowledge of research findings that dispel existing myths surrounding visiting (Annotated Bibliography: 3, 6; Suggested Readings: 20). Nurses report that open visiting practices take extra time, cause delays, and make it difficult to concentrate on delivery of patient care (Annotated Bibliography: 3; Other References: 17, 81). Nurses who feel technically competent are likely to be more comfortable interacting with family members at the bedside than will nurses who are learning psychomotor skills necessary to care for critically ill patients (Suggested Readings: 14, 15; Other References: 81, 83). Second, nurses with high levels of empathy (able to form an accurate perception of the patient's and family's world and to communicate this understanding to the patient and family) have a greater ability to assess family members' needs accurately so that visiting hours start on time, they have frequent access to the patient, and visiting hours are changed for special conditions (Other References: 34).

Nurses need also to be competent in crisis intervention—able to listen actively, reduce anxiety, and diffuse those who may be angry and upset. This requires therapeutic communication to promote discussion of what the patient and family members know, to clarify misconceptions, and to reflect back to them what has been voiced. Competency in observing and vocalizing nonverbal cues of patients and families is also important (Other References: 5). An intervention checklist for initial (Appendix 3-D) and subsequent visits can help prompt busy staff to ask appropriate questions that communicate the importance of facilitating interaction between patient and family (Other References: 79). Nurses must also be competent in modeling for families how to interact with their loved one, to talk with and touch their loved one, to look past the machines and tubes, and to sit at the bedside.

Nurses need to be competent in making referrals for family members, patients, and themselves when they find it difficult to manage the interface between technology and humanism. Daily confrontation with the wide variety of emotions of patients and families is a challenge and may necessitate use of support services to meet identified needs. Providing processes for nurses to problem solve in specific situations and to deal with the emotions associated with facilitating family-patient interaction is extremely important (Other References: 64). These processes may take the form of support groups, consultation with clinical nurse specialists and chaplains, and use of innovations to prepare family members for visiting (eg, what questions to ask, how to participate in decision making) (Suggested Readings: 15).

For nurses to achieve these competencies, they must be afforded the opportunity to do the following:

1. Learn the research-based knowledge on visiting.
2. Clarify their values regarding incorporation of family members into care delivery.
3. Have discussions with their peers, other disciplines, and patients and family members who have undergone a critical care experience to arrive at consensus of what the visiting practice guidelines will be for their unit.
4. Disseminate the practice guidelines to appropriate multidisciplinary colleagues.
5. Post environmental cues and signs that are congruent with the practice guideline.
6. Receive ongoing administrative support for making research-based practice changes.

For many nurses, a turning point from excluding to including families in critical care practice is the personal experience of having a relative or loved one hospitalized in a critical care unit (Annotated Bibliography: 1).

Child Visitation in the Adult and Neonatal Intensive Care Unit

Use of the FCVI requires that staff know the developmental levels of children, use developmentally appropriate actions with various age groups of children, and be alert for the typical behaviors children display when under stress. Developmental tasks, typical problems of each age group, stress behaviors, and suggested actions are summarized in Appendix 3-E. Nurses must also be competent in active listening, anticipatory guidance, and fostering interaction among family members. As when intervening with adults, staff must be competent in role modeling touch and encouraging appropriate communication between the patient and child.

Some institutions recommend use of a health screening form (Appendix 3-F) and health screening guidelines (Appendix 3-G) when facilitating visits by children in the ICU. Contact your hospital epidemiology or infection control program for your institution's guidelines.

ETHICAL CONSIDERATIONS

Adult Critical Care Unit

The major ethical consideration is continuing rigid restrictive visiting practices when there is sufficient evidence to demonstrate that this is not the best practice for critically ill patients and their family members. A second consideration is the need to support and coach nursing staff, who are uncomfortable interacting with family members in the face of complex physiological care, to grow professionally in this component of their practice.

Child Visitation in the Adult and Neonatal Intensive Care Unit

The major ethical consideration for children visiting is allowing the child a choice. The decision for a child to visit in the adult or neonatal ICU should be mutual between the nonhospitalized adult (adult ICU) or parent (NICU) and the child. For children and parents who decide not to visit, the following strategies are available (Suggested Readings: 9):

- Read a book designed for children (an example for siblings is *The Frogs Have A Baby, A Very Small Baby* by Jerri Oehler).
- Encourage the child to send photos, colored pictures, or other appropriate items that can be displayed at the patient's bedside.
- Have the child read a story or talk to the critically ill baby or adult family member via audiotape recorder to be played at the bedside.
- Photograph or videotape the parent or nonhospitalized adult family member visits and share them with the child while explaining what is being seen and heard.
- In the neonatal ICU, have staff provide baby's footprints, handprints, or lock of hair to the child.
- Encourage parents to tell the child that you love him or her.
- Plan special activities with the child away from the hospital.
- Give honest, simple updates on the patient's condition.
- Provide consistent caretakers for the child, preferably in the child's home.
- Eat meals as a family daily, if possible.
- Reassure the child that the NICU baby's condition is not his or her fault.
- Discuss with the child the hospitalized adult's illness in simple terms and reassure the child that the illness is not his or her fault, as appropriate.
- Have the child color a picture or write a story about the critical care hospitalization, and use it as a focus of discussion.
- Hold and hug the child.
- Acknowledge your own feelings to the child in simple terms.
- Maintain as much of the normal routine in the child's life as possible.

COMPLICATIONS

Adult Critical Care Unit

A major potential complication with less restrictive visiting is easier access to critical care units and subsequent related violent acts to a patient or staff member. Less restricted visiting, however, does not mean free access to all patients by any family member (Other References: 32; Suggested Readings: 15).

Other potential complications include disruptive behaviors (eg, incessant talking, moving or manipulating equipment) and unexpected emotional (eg, extreme anxiety) and physiological reactions (eg, lightheadedness, fainting) of family members during interactions with the patient. Steps to minimize these potential complications include preparing family members for visits, particularly the first visit; model-

ing appropriate interactions between the patient and family member (eg, hand holding); educating family members about expected behaviors; reinforcing the importance of not moving or manipulating equipment without permission and guidance of staff; and preparing the patient care area for family members (eg, providing a chair at the bedside). The nurse should also monitor family members for cues indicating extreme anxiety or physiological changes and intervene by escorting them from the bedside or providing a chair. Family members who experience extreme emotional or physiological sequelae during the visit benefit from one-on-one counseling to discuss and resolve issues contributing to their response. Family members should also be instructed to refrain from visiting if they have a communicable illness (Suggested Readings: 14, 15, 17).

Special consideration is important for the critically ill patient who may have an episode of acute decompensation while the family is at the bedside. Family members will generally leave the bedside if asked during such episodes while others may want to stay. Because the physiological stability of the patient is the first priority, staff need a mechanism to call someone (eg, chaplain, another staff member, volunteer) to be with family members at the bedside if they chose to stay. Similarly, if family members are asked to leave, it is important that they have a support system in the waiting area and that staff discuss the incident with the family members when the patient has stabilized (Suggested Readings: 15).

Child Visitation in the Adult and Neonatal Intensive Care Unit

Hazards to children who visit are that the child (1) may dislike what is seen during the visit; (2) may have an increase in undesirable feelings and behaviors, such as increased upset or anger; or (3) could find the visit too overwhelming, perhaps causing lightheadedness or fainting. As with adults visiting in the adult critical care unit, these potential complications can be minimized by proper preparation of the child and nonhospitalized adult family member. Additionally, children who choose not to visit should not be coerced into visiting to please a nonhospitalized adult family member. Lastly, all children should be screened for communicable illness to decrease the risk of infection transmission.

FUTURE RESEARCH

Adult Critical Care Unit

Multisite, randomized, controlled trials are needed to test interventions that promote proximity of critically ill patients and their family members. Most of the evidence for less restricted visiting is from descriptive or quasi-experimental studies. More studies with culturally diverse populations are also needed to determine if visiting preferences differ by culture and the type of visiting practices that best meet the needs of various cultures. Visiting preferences of distinct age groups and the impact on patient outcomes of promoting proximity among family members need more intensive investigation.

Child Visitation in the Adult and Neonatal Intensive Care Unit

Large multisite studies with culturally diverse populations are needed to test the FCVI. Studies examining the longer-term effects of this intervention are also needed. Interviewing family members in their home about the effects of the FCVI would be helpful to determine the impact on coping strategies used by children outside the hospital environment. The impact of this intervention on patients is not well understood and needs further exploration.

General

More experimental or quasi-experimental studies are needed to test strategies for assisting nurses to develop positive attitudes and increase their knowledge about providing family-centered care, including visiting. These studies need to include a focus on the novice nurse—determining and evaluating techniques and tools to provide the knowledge and skills of therapeutic visitation necessary to optimally involve the family in the coordination of the patient's care. Studies are also needed to explicate the relationships among (1) the expectations and attitude of critical care nurse managers, (2) unit culture that promotes family-centered care, (3) staff behaviors and attitudes regarding family-centered care, and (4) intermediate and long-term outcomes of critically ill patients and family members.

SUGGESTED READINGS

In addition to the references in the annotated bibliography, the following will help provide practices that promote interactions among critically ill patients and their family members.

1. Consolvo CA. Siblings in the NICU. *Neonat Netw.* 1987; 5:7-12.
2. Johnson DL. Preparing children for visiting parents in the adult ICU. *Dimens Crit Care Nurs.* 1994;13:153-165.
3. Krapohl GL. Visiting hours in the adult intensive care unit: using research to develop a system that works. *Dimens Crit Care Nurs.* 1995;14:245-258.
4. LaMontagne LL. Three coping strategies used by school-age children. *Pediatr Nurs.* 1984;10(1):25-28.
5. Lazure LLA. Strategies to increase patient control of visiting. *Dimens Crit Care Nurs.* 1997;16:11-19.
6. Lewandowski LA. Needs of children during the critical illness of a parent or sibling. *Crit Care Clin North Am.* 1992;4:573-585.
7. Marfell JA, Garcia JS. Contracted visiting hours in the coronary care unit. A patient-centered quality improvement project. *Nurs Clin North Am.* 1995;30:87-97.
8. Molter NC. Families are not visitors in the critical care unit. *Dimens Crit Care Nurs.* 1994;13:2-3.
9. Montgomery LA, Kleiber C, Nicholson A, Craft-Rosenberg M. A research-based sibling visitation program for the neonatal ICU. *Crit Care Nurse.* 1997; 17(2);29-40.
10. Moseley MJ, Jones AM. Contracting for visitation with families. *Dimens Crit Care Nurs.* 1991;10:365-371.
11. Osborn MA, Downer L. Making your case. Using research to change policy. *Am J Nurs.* 1994;94(suppl): 21-26.
12. Poole EL. The visiting needs of critically ill patients and their families. *J Post Anesth Nurs.* 1992;7:377-386.
13. Shonkwiler MA. Sibling visits in the pediatric intensive care unit. *Crit Care Q.* 1985;8(1):67-72.
14. Tee N, Struthers C. It's time to change visiting policies in critical care units. *Can Nurse.* 1995;91(11):22-27.
15. Titler MG, Bombei C, Schutte DL. Developing family-focused care. *Crit Care Nurs Clin North Am.* 1995;7: 375-386.
16. Titler MG, Nicholson A, Montgomery LA, et al. Child visitation in adult critical care units. In: Funk SG, Tornquist EM, Champagne MT, Wiese RA, eds. *Key Aspects of Caring for the Acutely Ill.* New York, NY: Springer Publishing Co; 1995:256-267.
17. Titler MG, Walsh SM. Visiting critically ill adults. Strategies for practice. *Crit Care Nurs Clin North Am.* 1992;4:623-632.
18. Damboise C, Cardin, S. Family-centered critical care. How one unit implemented a plan. *Am J Nurs.* 2003; 103(6):56AA-56EE.
19. Giuliano KK, Giuliano AJ, Bloniasz E, Quirk PA, Wood J. A quality-improvement approach to meeting the needs of critically ill patients and their families. *Dimens Crit Care Nurs.* 2000;19(1):30-34.
20. Roland P, Russell J, Richards KC, Sullivan SC. Visitation in critical care: processes and outcomes of a performance improvement initiative. *J Nurs Care Qual.* 2001;15(2):18-26.
21. Slota M, Shearn D, Potersnak K, Haas L. Perspectives on family-centered, flexible visitation in the intensive care unit setting. *Crit Care Med.* 2003;31(5):S362-S366.

CLINICAL RECOMMENDATIONS

The rating scale for the Level of Recommendation ranges from I to VI, with levels indicated as follows: I, manufacturer's recommendations only; II, theory based, no research data to support recommendations; recommendations from expert consensus group may exist; III, laboratory data only, no clinical data to support recommendations; IV, limited clinical studies to support recommendations; V, clinical studies in more than 1 or 2 different populations and situations to support recommendations; VI, clinical studies in a variety of patient populations and situations to support recommendations.

Period of Use	Recommendation	Rationale for Recommendation	Level of Recommendation	Supporting References	Comments
Selection of Patients	Adult critically ill patients and their family members (≥ 14 years of age). (For children < 14 years of age see "Protocol for Children as Visitors in Adult and Neonatal Critical Care Units." See also "Protocol for Family Pet Visiting and Animal-assisted Activities and Therapy.")	Facilitating interaction between patient and family members is one component of family-centered critical care practice.	VI: Clinical studies in a variety of patient populations and situations to support recommendations	See Other References: 29 See Suggested Readings: 15, 17	
		Proximity ("the quality or state of being near or close") is consistently rated among the 10 most important needs of family members. The need "to see my relative frequently" is ranked first among visiting needs.		See Other References: 24, 30, 64, 77	
		Critically ill patients are part of a family system. What affects one member also affects the others. Critical illness contributes to family disorganization that goes beyond the CCU.		See Annotated Bibliography: 2	
Application and Use	*Family and Patient Assessment* Ask patients their preferences for: • who visits • length and frequency of visits • time of visits • unplanned visits Document information on plan of care.	Nurses' perceptions are sometimes incongruent with perceptions of patients and family members. Thus, it is important to understand the proximity needs from their perspective.	VI: Clinical studies in a variety of patient populations and situations to support recommendations	See Annotated Bibliography: 7 See Other References: 1, 16, 17, 34, 72, 74, 78, 82, 83 See also Leske JS, *Family Needs and Interventions in the Acute Care Environment* [Protocols for Practice]	If patient is unable to respond, ask a designated family member.

Period of Use	Recommendation	Rationale for Recommendation	Level of Recommendation	Supporting References	Comments
Application and Use *(cont.)*	*Family and Patient Assessment (cont.)*				
	Implement an individualized plan for visiting based on patient and family member preferences.	Visiting preferences differ by: • patient characteristics of age, degree of extroversion, socioeconomic status, and severity of illness • type of critical care unit (eg, MICU, SICU) • perceived stress of being in a critical care setting	VI: Clinical studies in a variety of patient populations and situations to support recommendations	See Other References: 5, 17, 59, 72, 74, 77, 83 See Suggested Readings: 8	Patients expect that nurses will help families to be sensitive to the patient's condition and adjust visiting practices accordingly.
	Prepare family members for visit, especially before the first visit. Consider using: • written guidelines • information or education books • videotapes • CD-ROM • interactive computer programs • photos or graphic illustrations • support group • one-on-one counseling During the presurgery phase, prepare patients and families for post-surgical visiting in cases where an ICU stay is expected. Consider using: • written guidelines • information/ education books • videotapes • tour of the unit	Family members who are prepared or educated about what to expect in the critical care unit tend to be more knowledgeable and satisfied, have more positive coping behaviors, and be less anxious than those who are not prepared for visiting.	V: Clinical studies in more than 1 or 2 different patient populations and situations to support recommendations	See Suggested Readings: 12, 15, 18, 19 See Other References: 20, 53, 61, 63, 79	
	Provide mechanisms for patients to assume control over their visits (eg, red and green lights; red and green flags).	Families are less hostile, depressed, and apprehensive and develop trust for health care providers when presence at the bedside is controlled by patient and family rather than the nurse.		See Annotated Bibliography: 4 See Other References: 6, 80 See Suggested Readings: 7, 10, 15	Care must be taken to avoid insisting that patients assume control because they may feel burdened rather than relieved.

Period of Use	Recommendation	Rationale for Recommendation	Level of Recommendation	Supporting References	Comments
Application and Use *(cont.)*	*Family and Patient Assessment (cont.)*				
	Offer to set up a patient-centered contract for visiting.	Contracts facilitate consistency in visiting among nurses for a specified patient and provide a sense of control for the patient (see example in Appendix B).			
Visiting Presence	Promote family members at the bedside as frequently as possible. Incorporate family members in provision of care, if agreed to by patient and family member.	Interaction between patients and family members promotes communication, enhances information exchange, increases family satisfaction, and has beneficial influences on patient outcomes.	VI: Clinical studies in a variety of patient populations and situations to support recommendations	See Annotated Bibliography: 1 See Suggested Readings: 17, 20 See Other References: 59, 61, 72, 79, 83	Encourage families also to get adequate rest and to eat appropriately.
		Families who are at the bedside are more likely to have needs met than they are with restricted visiting.			
		Discussions between nurses and family members help reduce family members' anxiety.			
		Involving family members in direct patient care may help decrease anxiety and feelings of powerlessness for some families.			
	Role model patient-family member interaction (touch, talking).	Family members may not know what they can touch, what they can say, or what they should do.		See Suggested Readings: 15 See Other References: 63	
	Explain condition of the patient and presence or absence of equipment.	Family members' anxiety is reduced if they know why equipment is gone and what it means for the patient.		See Other References: 16, 78 See Suggested Readings: 15	
	Provide written information, videos, or computer programs about visiting, unit environment, and hospital environment.	Families need concrete information, especially early in the ICU when their anxiety is high.		See Suggested Readings: 15, 18, 19 See Other References: 61, 79, 80	
	Refer family members for psychological, social, financial, and physical/health assistance as needed.	This is a high stress time. Families cope in a variety of ways and may need additional help coping with this experience.		See Annotated Bibliography: 2 See Other References: 8, 22, 24, 35, 64	

Period of Use	Recommendation	Rationale for Recommendation	Level of Recommendation	Supporting References	Comments
Visiting Presence *(cont.)*	Provide a mechanism for family members to stay "connected" with the patient when they leave the area (eg, beepers, cell phones, unit phone number).	Families receive a clear message that it is permissible and possible to leave the unit but still be in communication with staff.		See Other References: 20	
	Consider instituting a family education program on family-centered critical care (eg, video, written booklet, computer program).	Educational programs and helping families know what to expect reduce their stress and increase the frequency of their needs being met.	IV: Limited clinical studies to support recommendations	See Other References: 23, 53, 61	
	Adopt a unit philosophy of family-centered critical care practice, abolish restricted visiting policies and practices, and achieve unit consensus on a visiting practice guideline.	Restricted visiting in ICU is based on tradition, not science. Restricting patient-family interaction to short periods and terminating interactions prematurely contribute to adverse psychological and hemodynamic responses of critically ill patients. Presence of family members at the bedside may contribute to reducing ICPs.	VI: Clinical studies in a variety of patient populations and situations to support recommendations	See Annotated Bibliography: 4, 5, 6 See Other References: 4, 7, 15, 38, 40, 46, 59, 60, 65, 69, 74, 75 See Suggested Readings: 18, 19, 20	This is a process of planned change that incorporates helping staff change their beliefs and attitudes about visiting.
	Options to restricted visiting are: • flexible • by contract • patient controlled • structured • inclusive • open • individualized (See "General Description" for definitions.)	Patients and families prefer flexible, non-rigid visiting practices. Less restricted visiting results in increased family satisfaction and more needs of family members consistently met. Family visits are no more stressful than routine critical care nursing practice. When visiting policies are restrictive, some nurses bend the rules; families then view access to the patient as dependent on the ability to please staff. Conflicts among visitors and nurses may arise when nurses allow flexible visiting hours when a restrictive visiting policy is in place.		See Annotated Bibliography: 6, 7 See Suggested Readings: 21 See Other Readings: 48, 55, 59, 61, 72, 74, 83	

Period of Use	Recommendation	Rationale for Recommendation	Level of Recommendation	Supporting References	Comments
Visiting Presence *(cont.)*	Signs and environmental cues should be consistent with visiting guideline. Signs should reflect inclusion rather than exclusion.	Visitors receive mixed messages when a sign is posted outlining one type of visiting when another type of visiting is practiced. Overbearing signs placed at entrances to ICUs only contribute to family members' sense of powerlessness and anxiety at times of high stress.		See Suggested Readings: 17	
Ongoing Monitoring	Monitor patient and family responses during and after visits or interactions.	Individual patient variability in hemodynamic and psychological response to patient-family interaction is expected.	VI: Clinical studies in a variety of patient populations and situations to support	See Annotated Bibliography: 4, 5 See Other References: 46, 65, 74, 75	
	Decisions to limit or shorten visiting based on adverse hemodynamic response of patients should be made after the first 10-15 minutes.	Increases in HR and BP usually occur initially and then decline after the first 10-15 minutes. Interactions that are concluded naturally are more likely to result in return of cardiovascular responses to baseline than are interactions concluded prematurely.			
	Monitor family members' verbal and non-verbal response to visiting, especially early in the critical care experience. Refer to others for help as needed.	Family members who become extremely anxious, fearful, or withdrawn during visiting may need assistance in coping with the experience.		See Other References: 64	
	Monitor family vigilance at the hospital in relation to patient's severity of illness. If it is incongruent, assess further their: • understanding of the patient's status • previous experiences with ICUs • unique religious or cultural beliefs • unresolved feelings of guilt associated with past events			See Other References: 24 See Suggested Readings: 15	
	Monitor family members' energy level, fatigue, and physical self-care. Encourage	Families tend to sleep less, change their eating habits, consume more over-the-counter		See Annotated Bibliography: 2 See Other References: 78	

Period of Use	Recommendation	Rationale for Recommendation	Level of Recommendation	Supporting References	Comments
Ongoing Monitoring *(cont.)*	adequate sleep, nutrition, exercise, and breaks away from the hospital.	and prescription drugs, and deviate from normal family routines during the critical care hospitalization of a loved one.		See Suggested Readings: 15	
Quality Control Issues	Assure and facilitate competency in technical skills.	Nurses must perceive themselves as technically competent if family members are going to be at the bedside during care delivery. Less experienced nurses report aversion to being observed by visitors while providing patient care. The more competent the nurse, the more important visitors are perceived to be.	IV. Limited clinical studies to support recommendations.	See Suggested Readings: 15 See Other References: 81, 83	
	Assist nurses in changing negative attitudes and beliefs about families. Provide sessions to clarify values: • Reports and stories of ICU patients and families • Role playing • Case scenarios	Interventions to assist nurses in caring for patients and families must begin with changing negative attitudes and beliefs about families of critically ill patients.	V: Clinical studies in more than 1 or 2 different patient populations and situations to support recommendations	See Annotated Bibliography: 1, 3 See Other References: 21, 71 See Suggested Readings: 11, 14, 15,	
	Discuss myths and realities of the effect of family interactions on patients.	Nurses need to increase their research-based understanding of patient-family interaction.		See Suggested Readings: 20 See Other References: 48	
	Provide support for nurses who facilitate patient-family interaction: • Ongoing support group to deal with emotions • Problem-solving group to manage recurrent problems • Team members to be role models and to provide assistance with family visitation Provide feedback to staff regarding their interactions with patients and family members. Disseminate new scientific information to staff.	Nurses report that providing patient-family interactions is difficult and stressful.		See Suggested References: 18	

PROTOCOL FOR CHILDREN AS VISITORS IN ADULT AND NEONATAL CRITICAL CARE UNITS

Period of Use	Recommendation	Rationale for Recommendation	Level of Recommendation	Supporting References	Comments
Selection of Patients	Children ages 3-13 years who meet health and communicable disease screening criteria. Children with a positive history or assessment may be restricted from visiting (see Appendixes F and G for a sample screening form and guidelines).	Children under 3 years are not able to interpret cognitive cues clearly. Children 14 and over are often viewed as an "adult" for purposes of visiting by many institutions and thus are not typically restricted from visiting.	V: Clinical studies in more than 1 or 2 different patient populations and situations to support recommendations	See Other References: 3, 25, 33, 56, 68 See Suggested Readings: 9	This protocol may also be used with adolescents 14-17 years of age.
Application and Use	*Previsit Phase* 1. Explain the program; review benefits and risks of the visits with parent and child (dependent on age).	The decision for the child to visit is up to the individual family, with both child and parent having a voice, after the nursing staff have provided education and information. Often the situation imagined by the child is much more distressing than visiting their ill or injured family member.	V: Clinical studies in more than 1 or 2 different patient populations and situations to support recommendations	See Other References: 2, 33, 53, 54, 65, 67, 68, 71, 78 See Suggested Readings: 6, 9	The "dose" of this intervention may be altered to meet individual needs. For instance, as the child makes more visits to the critically ill sibling or adult, the time and amount of preparatory information provided may be reduced.
	Check with the parent to determine if the child has been asked if a visit is desired and agreed on. Schedule a visit time.	Children who are coerced or persuaded to visit when they do not want to may have adverse experiences that also are distressing for patient and other family members. (See "Ethical Considerations" for alternative actions if the child decides not to visit.)			If a child is distressed during the visit, additional debriefing with child and parental counseling may be necessary. Preparatory time for subsequent visits may need to be increased.
	2. Explore with the parent what the child knows about the critically ill adult or neonate patient: • What has the child been told? • What has child already seen or heard? • Have there been any notable behavior changes since the critical care hospitalization?				Additional resources available from University of Iowa Hospitals and Clinics Department of Nursing: • *Sibling Visitation in Special Care Nurseries* (1:23-min video for children) • Sibling visitation brochure

Period of Use	Recommendation	Rationale for Recommendation	Level of Recommendation	Supporting References	Comments
Application and Use *(cont.)*	*Previsit Phase (cont.)* Confirm that the parent will accompany the child to the bedside.				• *Helping Children Cope with the Intensive Care Unit* by Simone L. Hughes (parents and nurses to use with children visiting in adult ICU) • *Intensive Care Informational Book* by Simone L. Hughes (for children visiting in adult ICU)
	3. Check to be sure patient is stable and no procedures are scheduled.				
	4. Complete health communicable disease screening.	To decrease risk of infection transmission		See Other References: 14, 17, 20, 65	See Health Screening Form (Appendix F) and accompanying Guidelines (Appendix G) for action.
	Immediately Before the Visit				
	1. Meet with child and confirm desire to visit (eg, "Do you want to visit today?").	Children have the ability to understand difficult situations if explanations are provided in a developmentally appropriate manner.		See Suggested Readings: 6	
	2. Explain, using developmentally appropriate terms and actions, why the patient is in the hospital, what will happen during visit, and what the child might see, hear, and feel during the visit.				See Appendix E.
	3. Explain what equipment might be seen and how this is helping the patient.				
	4. Encourage the child to touch, stroke, and "talk" to the patient.				
	5. Prepare the patient and immediate environment for the visit: • Linen clean • Extraneous equipment away from the bedside • Privacy from other patients				

Period of Use	Recommendation	Rationale for Recommendation	Level of Recommendation	Supporting References	Comments
Application and Use *(cont.)*	*Immediately Before the Visit (cont.)*				
	This may be done by another nurse.				
	6. Assist the child to wash hands. Instruct parent to wash hands.				
	7. Hold child to put on mask and gown—no gloves (follow institution protocol).				Use of mask and gown differs by institution.
	During the Visit				
	1. Accompany the parent and child to the bedside.				
	2. Remain with parent and child during visit.				
	3. Continue to explain the appearance of the patient, encourage touch, explain equipment, monitor child's response, and facilitate conversation.				
	4. Watch for cues that the child is ready to leave the bedside and help bring the visit to a close. Most visits last 10-20 minutes.				
	Following the Visit				
	1. The nurse talks with child and parent about the visit:				A private area facilitates this discussion.
	• "Tell me about the visit."				If the child exhibits unusual behavior that the nurse is unable to manage, additional personnel resources should be called (eg, clinical nurse specialist; child development specialist; social worker, pastoral services; support personnel).
	• "How do you feel?"				
	• "Do you have any questions?" Nonverbal expression of the experience can also be facilitated (eg, color a picture; write a story) and serve as a focal point for discussion.				

Period of Use	Recommendation	Rationale for Recommendation	Level of Recommendation	Supporting References	Comments
Application and Use *(cont.)*	*Following the Visit (cont.)*				
	2. Encourage the parent to talk with the child about the visit after they leave the hospital. Instruct the parent about providing ongoing support for the child (eg, maintaining a sense of normalcy; keeping similar routines, habits, etc.; providing simple, honest updates about the critically ill patient).				
	3. Encourage the parent and child to arrange a subsequent visit, if desired.				
Ongoing Monitoring	Monitor child behavior and provide developmentally appropriate explanations.	Child may have questions during and after the visit.	V: Clinical studies in more than 1 or 2 different patient populations and situations to support recommendations	See Other References: 33, 68, 70 See Suggested Readings: 1, 2, 6, 9	
	Set limits on disruptive behavior at the bedside.				
	Watch for verbal and behavioral cues that the child wants to leave the bedside.				
	Monitor patient's response (BP, HR, dysrhythmia, oxygenation) before, during, and after the visit.				
	Instruct parent to continue support of child and ongoing monitoring of visit experience.				
Prevention of Complications	Use Health and Communicable Screening Form (Appendix F) and Guidelines (Appendix G) for child to prevent transmission of infection.		VI: Clinical studies in a variety of patient populations and situations to support recommendations	See Other References: 39, 66, 76	
	Minimize adverse behavior or feelings of the child: • Use developmentally appropriate communication (verbal, nonverbal).	Facilitating visiting of children in ICUs is a structured intervention with specific actions before, during, and after visiting.		See Other References: 33, 68, 70 See Suggested Readings: 9, 13	Encourage adequate rest and nourishment of the child before visiting.

Period of Use	Recommendation	Rationale for Recommendation	Level of Recommendation	Supporting References	Comments
Prevention of Complications *(cont.)*	• Prepare child. • Have child participate in decision whether to visit. • Accompany child to bedside. • Provide proper debriefing. Minimize patient complications by asking if patient wants child to visit.				
Quality Control Issues	Provide readily accessible materials necessary for this intervention to be carried out by staff (eg, make a "child visitation" tray with all of the necessary materials). Educate staff about the facilitated child visitation intervention with periodic updates. Provide a form for family to provide feedback on how to improve the FCVI program.	Facilitating children visiting in an ICU requires developmentally appropriate actions before, during, and following the visit.	VI: Clinical studies in a variety of patient populations and situations to support recommendations	See Suggested Readings: 2, 6, 9, 13 See Other References: 68, 70	

ANNOTATED BIBLIOGRAPHY

1. Chesla CA. Reconciling technologic and family care in critical-care nursing. *Image J Nurs Sch.* 1996;28:199-204.

Study Sample

The sample was 130 nurses from several hospitals caring for families in neonatal, pediatric, and adult critical care units. The majority of nurses (98%) held at least a baccalaureate degree. The 7 hospitals from which nurses were chosen included tertiary care teaching hospitals and community hospitals. The sample size was adequate.

Comparison Studied

This was a naturalistic, interpretive study of general critical care nursing done to describe nursing practice with families. There was no comparison group or intervention tested.

Study Procedures

Nurses were selected by their supervisors to represent varying levels of practice (advanced beginners to experts) and years of experience. Data were collected through interview with nurses in small groups with a focus on recent clinical practice. All nurses were interviewed 3 times. In addition, 48 nurses representative of all hospitals and levels of experience were observed in clinical practice for at least 2 hours on 3 occasions. This report focused on reporting the findings of 100 patient care transcribed narratives from the interviews. Transcribed interviews were coded using qualitative research methods.

Study Strengths and Weaknesses

This is a well-designed phenomenological study that details experiences of nurses in a naturalistic environment. Threats to validity are well addressed. The major weakness of this study is the exclusion of perceptions of family members.

Key Results

A range of practices emerged, including practices that focused on biophysical management of the patient as well as care that incorporated the family while at the same time addressing the complex technology of care. In situations that allowed flexibility in physical presence of family members with patients, expert nurses recognized and supported the family's role in care. This practice was often unpredictable, and when it did occur it often had outcomes that were a surprise to the nurse. However, direct family involvement with patients was far from the norm, particularly in adult critical care units. Some nurses could not see the value of including family in care and used multiple strategies to distance families. Other nurses provided expert, creative, and innovative care of families in the midst of continual demand for highly complex biophysical care delivery. For many nurses in the study, a turning point arose from personal experiences. Many nurses found that their perspective changed when a relative was hospitalized in a critical care unit and they had little access, inadequate information, and little influence on the plan of care. Opportunities to share these transformations with other critical care nurses might sensitize them to the importance of including family members in health care delivery.

Clinical Implications

There is a wide variation in using knowledge and family theory to guide practice. Nurses who are experts in family care and family therapy need to be introduced into critical care environments as consultants or educators in order to increase the overall skill level of nurses at the bedside.

2. Halm MA, Titler MG, Kleiber C, et al. Behavioral responses of family members during critical illness. *Clinical Nursing Research.* 1993;2: 414-437.

Study Sample

The sample consisted of 52 adult family members representing 48 families of patients admitted to a neonatal, pediatric, surgical, cardiac, or medical ICU at a large midwestern teaching hospital.

Comparison Studied

The purpose of this exploratory study was to describe the behavioral responses of adult family members to the critical care hospitalization of a loved one and to describe how stress responses change over the course of the critical care experience. Behavioral responses included self-reported changes in sleep, eating, and activity levels. Stress responses were increases or decreases in specific sleeping, eating, and activity behaviors.

Study Procedures

Behavioral responses of family members were measured by the self-report Iowa ICU Family Scale. The scale contains Likert-type items and open-ended questions to explore the 5 areas of sleep, eating, activity, family roles, and support systems. Family member self-reported information was collected each day during the first week of hospitalization and then weekly throughout the patient's ICU stay.

Key Results

Family members reported sleeping less with a poorer quality of sleep; consuming less nutritional food; increasing their use of cigarettes, alcohol, and over-the-counter and prescription medications; and spending the majority of their time talking, waiting, and visiting the patient. Stress was highest at the time of the ICU admission, began to plateau at day 6, and then dropped considerably by day 28.

Study Strengths and Weaknesses

The convenience sample is a study limitation, and the method used to understand changes in family member behaviors over time is a strength.

Clinical Implications

Assessment of family members shortly after critical care admission is essential to determine those at highest risk for stress and maladaptive coping and to intervene in order to help family members meet their needs. Sleep deprivation and fatigue are problems for family members, who may thus process limited amounts of information at one time and need information repeated. Hospitals should design areas adjacent to the critical care units that stock nutritious foods. Referrals to social workers, chaplains, clinical nurse specialists, or psychiatric nurses should also be considered for family members, particularly those whose loved one is at high risk.

3. **Kirchhoff KT, Pugh E, Calame RM, Reynolds N. Nurses' beliefs and attitudes toward visiting in adult critical care settings.** *Am J Crit Care.* **1993;2:238-245.**

Study Sample

Subjects were randomly selected from 5 ICUs in 4 hospitals in Utah and 3 ICUs in Ohio. The Utah sample consisted of 29 nurses employed in an adult ICU. Average age was 34 years and the majority were female (93%) and had a bachelor's degree (41.4%). The Ohio sample consisted of 41 nurses from an Ohio teaching hospital. Average age was 30.7 years and the majority (61%) held a bachelor's degree.

Comparison Studied

This study described the beliefs and attitudes of critical care nurses about the effects of visiting on patients, staff, and family. Nurses came from 2 different geographic locations and reported a variety of visiting policies in their units.

Study Procedures

A 20% sample of nurses was randomly selected from the schedule on the identified critical care units. Nurses needed to be an RN assigned to a day, day-night, or evening shift, and employed full- or part-time for at least 6 months in the ICU. Nurses were interviewed regarding their beliefs about visiting and given a questionnaire to assess their attitudes toward visiting. Results were analyzed by geographic location.

Key Results

The highest frequency of beliefs in each group was that limitations on visiting were important to prevent family members from staying longer than they should. About half (Utah, 45%; Ohio, 54%) of the nurses believed that the physiological effect of having visitors at the bedside was harmful. Beliefs about consequences of visiting on the unit were pri-

marily negative. Visiting was believed to make it difficult for the nurse to concentrate and feel in control of the situation, resulting in chaos, increased traffic, and delay in providing care. A positive belief was that inclusion of family enhances nursing care because of information transfer between family and care provider. The Ohio sample had consistently more positive attitudes than the Utah sample toward visiting. Effects of the consequences of visiting on family and unit were seen as predominately negative by most respondents.

Study Strengths and Weaknesses

Strengths of this study include random selection of subjects, multisite data collection, and integrating findings into a theoretical model that is clinically meaningful. Minor weaknesses include the varying sample size from the 2 sites, and reporting of steps taken to ensure the validity of interview data. This important study illustrates the need to change nurses' attitude and behavior regarding visiting practices.

Clinical Implications

Because beliefs and attitudes form behavior, these findings suggest that altering visiting policies will not alone be successful in providing family-centered care. Interventions to help nurses interact with families must be directed at changing negative attitudes and beliefs about families.

4. **Lazure LL, Baun MM. Increasing patient control of family visiting in the coronary care unit.** *Am J Crit Care.* **1995;4:157-164.**

Study Sample

The sample consisted of 60 subjects (randomly assigned to an experimental or a control group) from a midwestern metropolitan university hospital who were admitted to an 8-bed coronary care unit. Patients were relatively stable with the majority admitted for rule-out myocardial infarction. The experimental (n = 30) and control (n = 30) groups were equivalent on all demographic variables except race—there were more African Americans in the control than in the experimental group.

Comparison Studied

This randomized, controlled trial tested the efficacy of a patient-controlled visit timing device on the stress response (perceived control over visiting, HR, rhythm, premature ventricular contractions [PVCs], BP, salivary cortisol, finger temperature). Experimental group subjects used a patient-controlled access device to visiting (PCA-V) to signal potential visitors. Red and green lights outside the room indicated whether the visitor's presence was desired (green light) or not desired (red light). The control group interacted with visitors based on unit practice guidelines. The authors reported the unit policy as "Visiting regulations posted at the entrance limited visits to 30 minutes every 2 hours from 10 AM to noon, 2 to 4 PM, and 6 to 8 PM, but adherence to these posted regulations were rare."

Study Procedures

Heart rate and PVC incidence were measured by an arrhythmia monitoring system every 5 minutes from visit entry, during the first 20 minutes of visit, and at visit end. Blood pressure was measured using an automatic BP monitor that collected data every 6 minutes. Salivary cortisol was obtained 20 minutes into the first evening visit after 5 PM. Peripheral finger temperatures were collected every minute. Previsit and postvisit comfort, stress, and perceived control were assessed using vertical visual analog scales.

Key Results

Over time, perceived control of visits and rests between visits were greater, and HR and DBP were lower for subjects using the PCA-V device. The expected initial increase in BP and HR in response to visitor entry generally decreased within 10 minutes and returned to baseline by visit end in an unrestricted visiting environment. Patients had positive comments about use of the device.

Study Strengths and Weaknesses

This is a well-designed study that needs to be replicated in multiple sites using a more diverse sample. Potential limitations are the unknown standardization of visiting in the control group patients as posted visiting guidelines were not followed, and the transferability of the intervention to practice as the intervention is a product designed by the investigator that is not yet available for use. The device was tested in a unit that had private rooms, which may not be the case in some critical care settings. Despite these limitations, this is a very exciting study that tests an intervention that addresses ICU visitation.

Clinical Implications

Although further studies are needed to test this device with additional and more severely compromised critically ill patients, it holds great promise for the future. Placing control over visiting in the hands of patients when they are able to make such choices is an important strategy to facilitate interaction among patients and family members.

5. Schulte DA, Burrell LO, Gueldner SH. Pilot study of the relationship between heart rate and ectopy and unrestricted vs restricted visiting hours in the coronary care unit. *Am J Crit Care.* 1993;2:134-136.

Study Sample

The sample for this study was 25 visits to patients admitted to a coronary care unit for a cardiac condition (MI, chest pain). Thirteen visits occurred in the unrestricted visiting

policy group, and 12 visits occurred in the restricted visiting policy group. More subjects were diagnosed with an MI in the unrestricted than in the restricted visiting group.

Comparison Studied

The purpose of this pilot study was to determine the relationship between cardiac performance (HR, ectopy) and unrestricted versus restricted visiting hours in patients admitted to a critical care unit.

Study Procedures

One unit had restricted visiting (10 minutes at 6:00 and 9:00 AM, and 1:00, 5:00, and 8:30 PM; families were asked to leave during emergencies) and the second had unrestricted visiting. Heart rate and ectopy were measured before visitors arrived, 5 minutes after visitors arrived, and 1 to 5 minutes after the visitors left.

Key Results

Groups did not differ with respect to ectopy but did differ with respect to HR. Subjects in the unrestricted visiting group had significant declines in HR after visits, whereas heart rates of patients with restricted visits continued to increase.

Study Strengths and Weaknesses

A limitation of this study is the greater number of subjects in the unrestricted visiting group who were on more antidysrhythmic medications, which had an interactive effect with the unrestricted visiting intervention. A larger sample size is needed in the future. Despite these limitations, this pilot study was able to detect decline in HR when visits are unrestricted rather than terminated prematurely.

Clinical Implications

These findings suggest that premature termination of interaction between family members and patients has an adverse effect on heart rate.

6. Carlson B, Riegel B, Thomason T. Visitation. Policy versus practice. *Dimens Crit Care Nurs.* 1998;17(1):40-47.

Study Sample

Subjects were 882 nurses, representing all but 2 states within the United States, who cared for AMI patients during the first few days of hospitalization. Most subjects (83.6%) were members of the American Association of Critical Care Nurses (AACN), 89.9% worked in intensive or coronary care, 93.3% were female between the ages 31 and 40, 78.5% worked full-time, 94.1% were educated in the United States, 86.7% were certified in Advanced Cardiac Life Support and/or as a CCRN (50.6%), and 44.8% had a baccalaureate degree. Subjects had an average of 13.3 years experience as a nurse and 9.2 years experience as a critical care nurse. All sizes of hospitals were represented with 40.1% teaching hospitals.

Comparison Studied

This report describes current visiting practices and reasons for deviation from institutional policy. It is part of a descriptive study that examined practice among nurses caring for AMI patients.

Study Procedures

The results described in this article were derived from two specific items on visiting (one quantitative item, one qualitative item), included in a survey that consisted of 33 items and 14 demographic items. Surveys were mailed to a random sample of nurses who belonged to AACN and cared for AMI patients. Survey were also mailed to managers of critical care units, listed by the American Hospital Association, to be distributed to nurses caring for AMI patients. Return rate was 34.8%.

Key Results

Visitation policies included structured visiting times such as 10 minutes every 2 hours (53.5%), open visiting with some limitations by nurses (39.2%), totally open, free visiting allowed (3.8%), and visitation highly discouraged or limited (0.9%). Most nurses reported they always (14.4%) or sometimes (65.1%) personally deviated from unit policy. No significant differences were evident based on age, educational level, primary unit worked, AACN membership, or hospital size. The most frequently cited reason for deviating from the visiting policy was related to patient physiologic factors including patient condition or acuity (44.7%), critical, deteriorating, or dying condition (32.8%), patient stability (15.8%), do-not-resuscitate status (2.8%), and presence of chest pain (2.4%). Other reasons included family/visitor factors (25.8%), patient desires or needs (23.9%), patient situation or circumstances (14.1%), patient response to visiting (11.2%), and unit factors (3.1%).

Study Strengths and Weaknesses

This study was strengthened by the large sample size, 2 random sampling methods involving the entire United States, and the open-ended method of soliciting details. However, it was limited by having only 2 questions and by being part of a 33-item survey. Further, the investigators were unable to discern whether deviations from visitation policies were to liberalize or further restrict the visitation prescribed by unit policy. Potential bias concerns include the low response rate and having nurse managers distribute the surveys.

Clinical Implications

These findings suggest that visitation policies are being liberalized and that nurses are individualizing visiting. However, wide variability continues to be evident. This study provided insight into the factors that contribute to nursing

behaviors surrounding visitation in the intensive care environment. Further research utilizing qualitative methodologies would provide information about how and why nurses make family visitation decisions. Although it is not known whether nurses liberalized or further restricted family visitation related to these factors, these findings support that visiting policies need to consider the variability of needs and circumstances that exist in the critically ill population as well as consideration of the nurse's role as patient advocate and care coordinator.

7. Gonzales CE, Carroll DL, Elliott JS, Fitzgerald PA, Vallent HJ. Visiting preferences of patients in the intensive care unit and in a complex care medical unit. *Am J Crit Care.* 2004;13(3): 194-198.

Study Sample

Subjects were 31 adult patients in an intensive care unit and 31 adult patients in a complex care medical unit within a large academic medical center. Subjects included 36 men and 25 women, with a mean age of 61 years. All patients were alert and oriented with no known active psychiatric illness, able to speak English, in stable hemodynamic condition, and not intubated.

Comparison Studied

The purpose of this descriptive study was to describe patients' preferences for family visiting in an intensive care unit (ICU) and a complex care medical unit (CCMU); specifically, to measure the perceived benefits, stressors, and outcomes of family visiting and the preferences of patients from an ICU and a CCMU regarding visitors.

Study Procedures

The Patient's Perceptions of Visiting in the Hospital questionnaire was used to interview the patient and record responses during a structured interview while the patient was an inpatient. The questionnaire contains Likert-type items to explore stressors, benefits, and outcomes of visiting. Comments by the subject were written verbatim in the free text section.

Key Results

Patients rated visiting as a nonstressful experience because visitors offered moderate levels of reassurance, comfort, and calming effects. Patients did not perceive that visitors hindered rest or intensified pain. A stressor was worry about their visitors' traveling to visit them. Patients valued the fact that visitors can assist them in interpreting the information provided by health care providers and that visitors can provide information to help nurses understand a patient's personality and coping style. Patient preferences included unlimited visiting hours (37%), visitors only once a day (35%), visitors in the afternoon (50%), visiting to end at 8

PM (32%), and visitors restricted if a patient was experiencing signs or symptoms (22%). Patients preferred visits to be restricted when patients were unsure of the daily routine, were not feeling well, when family or visitor dynamics were not optimal, and in the early morning and late evening when resting. Patient desired limited visiting when procedures were scheduled or when speaking with their physicians. Patients preferred 3 visitors per visit, 3 (ICU) to 4 (CCMU) times a day, and a minimum age of visitors to be 14 (ICU) and 12 (CCMU) years.

Study Strengths and Weaknesses

This is a well-designed study. Generalizability of findings is limited because of the small sample size, the sample of patients may not reflect typical ICU patients, and use of 1 site for data collection.

Clinical Implications

Although patients expressed satisfaction with flexible visiting hours, patients did indicate times during which visitors should be restricted. These findings support the need for patients and nurses to communicate openly and to collaboratively devise a plan for visiting to best meet the needs of patients, visitors, and health care providers.

OTHER REFERENCES

1. Artinian NT. Selecting a model to guide family assessment. *Dimens Crit Care Nurs.* 1994;14(1):5-12.
2. Azarnoff P. Parents and siblings of pediatric patients. *Curr Probl Pediatr.* 1984;14:1-40.
3. Baker C, Nieswidomy R, Arnold W. Nursing interventions for children with a parent in the intensive care unit. *Heart Lung.* 1988;17:441-446.
4. Bay EJ, Kupferschmidt B, Opperwall BJ, Speer J. Effect of family visit on patients' mental status. *Focus on Crit Care.* 1988;15(1):11-16.
5. Boykoff S. Visitation needs reported by patients with cardiac disease and their families. *Heart Lung.* 1986;15:573-578.
6. Brannon P, Brady A, Gailey A. Visitation in the CCU: from "rules" to contracts. *Nurs Management.* 1990;21:64M-64P.
7. Bruya M. Planned periods of rest in the intensive care unit: nursing activities and intracranial pressure. *J Neurosurg Nurs.* 1981;13:184-194.
8. Bunn T, Clarke A. Crisis intervention: an experimental study of a brief period of counseling on the anxiety of relatives of seriously injured or ill hospital patients. *Br J Med Psychol.* 1979;52:191-195.
9. Cohen MZ, Craft MJ, Titler MG. Families in critical care settings: where fear leads to silence. *Phenomenology and Pedagogy.* 1988;6(3):10-15.
10. Cohen MZ, Titler MG, Craft MJ. Validation of alterations in family processes: perceptions of critical care hospitalization. In: Carroll-Johnson RM, ed. *Classification of Nursing Diagnosis: Proceedings of the Eighth Conference.* Philadelphia, Pa: JB Lippincott; 1989:328-332.
11. Craft MJ. Siblings of hospitalized children: assessment and intervention. *J Pediatr Nurs.* 1993;8:289-297.
12. Craft MJ. Validation of responses reported by school-aged siblings of hospitalized children. *Children's Health Care.* 1986;15(1):6-13.
13. Dunkel J, Eisendrath S. Families in the intensive care unit: their effect on staff. *Heart Lung.* 1983;12:258-261.
14. Ferguson B. Preparing young children for hospitalization: a comparison of two methods. *Pediatrics.* 1979;64:656-664.
15. Guliano K, Guliano A. Cardiovascular responses to family visitation and nurse physical rounds. *Heart Lung.* 1992; 21:290-295.
16. Halm MA. Support and reassurance needs. *Crit Care Nurs Clin North Am.* 1992;4:633-643.
17. Halm M, Titler M. Appropriateness of critical care visitation: perceptions of patient, family members, nurses and physicians. *J Nurs Quality Assurance.* 1990;5(1):25-37.
18. Hamner JB. Visitation policies in the ICU: a time for change. *Crit Care Nurse.* 1990;10(1):48-49, 52-53.
19. Heater B. Nursing responsibilities in changing visiting restrictions in the intensive care unit. *Heart Lung.* 1985; 14:181-186.
20. Henneman EA, Cardin S. Need for information. *Crit Care Clin North Am.* 1992;4:615-621.
21. Hickey ML, Lewandowski M. Critical care nurses' role with families: a descriptive study. *Heart Lung.* 1988;17:670-676.
22. Hodovanic B, Reardon D, Reese W, Hedges B. Family crisis intervention program in the medical intensive care unit. *Heart Lung.* 1984;13:243-249.
23. Johnson PT. Critical care visitation: an ethical dilemma. *Crit Care Nurse.* 1988;8(6):72,75-78.
24. Johnson SK, Craft M, Titler M, et al. Perceived changes in adult family members' roles and responsibilities during critical illness. *Image J Nurs Sch.* 1995;27:238-243.
25. Johnstone M. Children visiting members of their family receiving treatment in ICUs: a literature review. *Intensive Crit Care Nurs.* 1994;10:289-292.
26. Kirchhoff K, Hansen CB, Fuller N. Open visiting in the ICU: a debate. *Dimens Crit Care Nurs.* 1985;4:296-306.
27. Kleiber C, Halm M, Titler M, et al. Emotional responses of family members during a critical care hospitalization. *Am J Crit Care.* 1994;3(1):70-76.
28. Leske JS. Family member interventions: research challenges. *Heart Lung.* 1991;20:391-393.
29. Leske JS. Needs of adult family members after critical illness: prescriptions for interventions. *Crit Care Clin North Am.* 1992;4:587-596.

30. Lust B. The patient in the ICU: a family experience. *Crit Care Quality.* 1984;6:49-57.

31. Maloney M, Ballard J, Hollister L, Shank M. A prospective, controlled study of scheduled sibling visits to a newborn intensive care unit. *J Am Acad Ped.* 1983; 22:565-570.

32. McClowry SG. Family functioning during a critical illness. *Crit Care Nurs Clin North Am.* 1992;4:559-564.

33. Montgomery LA. *Response in Preschool Children to the Hospitalization of a Newborn Sibling* [master's thesis]. Iowa City, Iowa: University of Iowa College of Nursing; 1988.

34. Murphy PA, Forrester DA, Price DM, Monaghan JF. Empathy of intensive care nurses and critical care family needs assessment. *Heart Lung.* 1992;21:25-30.

35. O'Keeffe B, Gilliss CL. Family care in the coronary care unit: an analysis of clinical specialist intervention. *Heart Lung.* 1988;17:191-198.

36. Owen J, Hammons M, Brooks B, Cain C, Smith I, Mann S. Changing visiting policy. *Dimens Crit Care Nurs.* 1988;7:369-373.

37. Stockdale LL, Hughes JP. Critical care unit visiting policies: a survey. *Focus Crit Care.* 1988;15:45-48.

38. Treloar DM, Nalli BJ, Guin P, Gary R. The effect of familiar and unfamiliar voice treatments on intracranial pressure in head injured patients. *J Neurosci Nurs.* 1991;23:295-299.

39. Umphenour J. Bacterial colonization in neonates with sibling visitation. *J Obstet Gynecol Neonatal Nurs.* 1980; 9:73-75.

40. Vanson SR, Katz BM, Krekeler K. Stress effects on patients in critical care units from procedures performed on others. *Heart Lung.* 1980;9:494-497.

41. West AM. Suggestions for healthcare providers in critical care units [letter]. *Heart Lung.* 1989;18:103-104.

42. Woellner DS. Flexible visiting hours in the adult critical care unit. *Focus Crit Care.* 1988;15:66-69.

43. Wolfer J, Visintainer M. Pediatric surgical patients and parents' stress responses and adjustment as a function of psychological preparation and stress point nursing care. *Nurs Res.* 1985;24:244-255.

44. Woolley N. Crisis theory: a paradigm of effective intervention with families of critically ill people. *J Adv Nurs.* 1990;15:1402-1408.

45. Younger SJ, Coulton C, Welton R, Juknialis B, Jackson DL. ICU visiting policies. *Crit Care Med.* 1984;12: 606-608.

46. Zetterlund J. An evaluation of visiting policies for intensive and coronary care units. In: Puffy M, Anderson M, Bergerson B, eds. *Current Concepts in Clinical Nursing.* St. Louis, Mo: CV Mosby; 1971:316-325.

47. Berwick D, Kotagal M. Restricted visiting hours in ICUs. Time to change. *JAMA.* 2004;292(6):736-737.

48. Chow SM. Challenging restricted visiting policies in critical care. *CACCN.* 1999;10(2):24-27.

49. Cullen L, Titler M, Drahozal R. Family and pet visitation in the critical care unit. *Crit Care Nurs.* 2003;23(5): 62-66.

50. Gottlieb JAK. Time to care: the evolution and meaning of family visiting policies in the intensive care unit. *Int J Hum Caring.* 2003;7(2):66-71.

51. Miracle VA. Critical care visitation. *Dimens Crit Care Nurs.* 2003;22(1):48-47.

52. Ramsey, P, Cathelyn J, Gugliotta B, Glenn LL. Restricted versus open ICUs. *Nurs Manage.* 2000;(January):42-44.

53. Chavez CW, Faber L. Effect of an education-orientation program on family members who visit their significant other in the intensive care unit. *Heart Lung.* 1987;16: 92-99.

54. Craft MJ, Cohen MZ, Titler M, DeHamer M. Experience in children of critically ill parents: a time of emotional disruption and need for support. *Crit Care Nurs Q.* 1993;16(3):64-71.

55. Craft MJ, Craft JL. Perceived changes in siblings of hospitalized children: a comparison of sibling and parent reports. *Child Health Care.* 1989;18:42-48.

56. Craft MJ, Wyatt N. Effect of visitation upon siblings of hospitalized children. *Matern Child Nurs J.* 1986; 47-59.

57. Craft MJ, Wyatt N, Sandell B. Behavior and feeling changes in siblings of hospitalized children. *Clin Pediatr.* 1985;24:374-378.

58. Frederickson K. Anxiety transmission in the patient with myocardial infarction. *Heart Lung.* 1989;18:17-22.

59. Frederickson K. Anxiety transmission in the patient with myocardial infarction. *Heart Lung.* 1989;18:17-22.

60. Fuller BF, Foster GM. The effects of family/friend visits vs staff interaction on stress/arousal of surgical intensive care patients. *Heart Lung.* 1982;11:457-463.

61. Henneman EA, McKenzie JB, Dewa CS. An evaluation of interventions for meeting the information needs of families of critically ill patients. *Am J Crit Care.* 1992; 3:85-93.

62. Hendrickson SL. Intracranial pressure changes and family presence. *J Neurosci Nurs.* 1987;19:14-17.

63. Holl RM. Role-modeled visiting compared with restricted visiting on surgical cardiac patients and family members. *Crit Care Nurs Q.* 1993;16(2):70-82.

64. Kleiber C, Montgomery LA, Craft-Rosenberg M. Information needs of siblings of critically ill children. *Child Health Care.* 1995;24:47-60.

65. Kleman M, Bickert A, Karpinski A, et al. Physiologic responses of coronary care patients to visiting. *J Cardiovasc Nurs.* 1993;7(3):52-62.

66. Kowba MD, Schwirian PM. Direct sibling contact and bacterial colonization in newborns. *J Obstet Gynecol Neonatal Nurs.* 1985;14:412-417.

67. Newman CB, McSweeney M. A descriptive study of sibling visitation. *Neonatal Netw.* 1990;9(4):27-31.

68. Nicholson AC, Titler MG, Montgomery LA, et al. Effects of child visitation in adult critical care units: A pilot study. *Heart Lung.* 1993;22:36-45.

69. Prins MM. The effect of family visits on intracranial pressure. *West J Nurs Res.* 1989;11:281-297.

70. Schwab F, Tolbert B, Bagnato S, Maisels MJ. Sibling visiting in a neonatal intensive care unit. *Pediatrics.* 1983;71:835-838.

71. Simon SK, Phillips K, Badalamenti S, Ohlert J, Krumberger J. Current practices regarding visitation policies in critical care units. *Am J Crit Care.* 1997;6:210-217.

72. Simpson T. Critical care patients' perceptions of visits. *Heart Lung.* 1991;20:681-688.

73. Simpson T. Visit preferences of middle-aged vs older critically ill patients. *Am J Crit Care.* 1993;2:339-345.

74. Simpson T, Shaver J. Cardiovascular responses to family visits in coronary care unit patients. *Heart Lung.* 1990;19:344-351.

75. Simpson T, Shaver J. A comparison of hypertensive and nonhypertensive coronary care patients' cardiovascular responses to visitors. *Heart Lung.* 1991;20:213-220.

76. Solheim K, Spellacy C. Sibling visitation: effects on newborn infection rates. *J Obstet Gynecol Neonatal Nurs.* 1988;18:43-48.

77. Stillwell SB. Importance of visiting needs as perceived by family members of patients in the intensive care unit. *Heart Lung.* 1984;13:238-242.

78. Titler MG, Cohen MZ, Craft MJ. Impact of adult critical care hospitalization: perceptions of patients, spouses, children, and nurses. *Heart Lung.* 1991;20:174-182.

79. Ward CR, Constancia PE, Kern L. Nursing interventions for families of cardiac surgery patients. *J Cardiovasc Nurs.* 1990;5(1):34-42.

80. Ziemann KM, Dracup K. Patient-nurse contracts in critical care: a controlled trial. *Prog Cardiovasc Nurs.* 1990;5(3):98-103.

81. Plowright CI. Intensive therapy unit nurses' beliefs about and attitudes towards visiting in three district general hospitals. *Intensive Crit Care Nurs.* 1998;14(6): 262-270.

82. Ramsey P, Cathelyn J, Gugliotta B, Glenn LL. Visitor and nurse satisfaction with a visitation policy change in critical care units. *Dimens of Crit Care Nurs.* 1999; 18(5):42-48.

83. Wong FY, Arthur DG. Hong Kong patients; experiences of intensive care after surgery: nurses' and patients' views. *Intensive Crit Care Nurs.* 2000;16(5): 290-303.

Family Assessment: Key Areas and Questions for Adults

PART I: PERCEPTION, EXPERIENCE, AND KNOWLEDGE OF FAMILY MEMBERS

1. Family perceptions
   A. What do you and other family members know about your loved one's condition?
   B. What was he or she doing before coming to the hospital? to the ICU?
   C. Can you tell me why your family member is in the ICU?
   D. What activities could he or she do before this happened?

2. Past experiences with ICUs
   A. Have you, another family member, or friend been a patient in an ICU? in this ICU? If yes, what was this experience like for you?
   B. What do you know about ICUs?

3. Health maintenance activities
   A. Do any family members have health problems we should know about?
   B. Do you or any other family members have special health care needs?
   C. Are family members eating properly? getting some rest? taking a break away from the ICU?

4. Knowledge of health care workers
   A. Has anyone explained the team of people that will be caring for your family member?
   B. Would you like me to write down the names of the physicians, nurses, and other people caring for your family member?

C. Would you be interested in setting up a daily information meeting with the doctor or nurse?
   D. Would you like the nurse caring for your family member to contact you at a specified time each day?

5. Knowledge of the unit policies and telephone numbers
   A. Has anyone explained unit practices regarding visiting, use of waiting areas, and calling to find out the condition of your family member?
   B. Did you receive our family orientation book?
   C. Have you been able to watch the video about our unit?
   D. Do you have the unit telephone number and waiting-room telephone number?
   E. Has anyone talked to you about our communication board?
   F. Do you have any questions for me?

PART II: PSYCHOSOCIAL FAMILY FUNCTIONS

1. Family constellation and roles
   A. What is your relationship to the patient?
   B. What other family members are present?
   C. Can you describe the roles and responsibilities of the patient and of each family member?
   D. Who will temporarily take over the patient's role?
   E. How many children, if any, does the patient have?

2. Family coping
   A. What have you and other family members done in the past to deal with stressful situations?
   B. How have other family members coped in the past with illness? with stress? with anxiety?
   C. Does the family view the patient's illness as a crisis?

D. Has the family experienced other recent losses, changes, or stressors?

E. What is the ability of the family to air concerns? to problem solve? to make decisions?

3. Economic and social resources

A. What are the family's economic resources? Do they have health care insurance?

B. What needs do you have for financial assistance?

C. What support systems are available to the family?

D. Are any family members interested in talking with a social worker, clergy, or clinical nurse specialist?

E. In the past, who has been supportive to the patient? to the family?

Source: Used with permission by the Family Intervention Research Team, University of Iowa Hospitals and Clinics and The University of Iowa College of Nursing, Iowa City, Iowa.

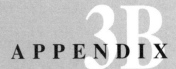

Sample Contract to Facilitate Adult Visiting

Hospital name: _____   Unit name: _____

Patient name: _____

Nurse completing contract: _____

A. What specific requests do you have about people visiting you while you are in the ICU?

1. What times during the day? _____

2. How long? _____

3. How many visitors at a time? _____

4. Are there any children you would like to have visit you?

   If yes, name and age: _____

5. Are there people you would NOT like to have visit you?

   _____

6. Do you rest better with ❑ or without ❑ family/visitors present? _____

   _____ (specify: family member/others?)

Comments: _____

B. Who should we call if you need someone?

Name: _____   Relationship: _____

Phone numbers: (work) _____   (home) _____

Name (alternate): _____   Relationship: _____

Phone numbers: (work) _____   (home) _____

C. Who is the family member that should receive daily updates on your condition?

Name: _____   Relationship: _____

Phone numbers: (work) _____   (home) _____

Best time of day to contact: _____

D. Who, if anyone, do you want to designate as a spokesperson for you?

E. Do you want a family member to participate in your care? No _____ Yes _____

Name: _____   Relationship: _____

Preferred time of day: _____

   Type of care activities:

   Bathing _____ Meals _____ Exercise _____

   Back rubs _____ Other _____

Patient signature (if able): _____

Family member signature: _____
(if patient unable to sign)

Nurse signature: _____

Date of original contract: _____   Revision date(s): _____

This form is only a sample. Changes should be made to fit individual unit practices and policies. For example, if visiting is available only at specified times, those times should be listed in A.1. Additional statements (eg, "Staff reserve the right to limit visitors based on status of the patient and overall status of the unit") may be added.

Source: Used with permission by the Family Intervention Research Team, University of Iowa Hospitals and Clinics and The University of Iowa College of Nursing, Iowa City, Iowa.

Topics to Consider for Inclusion in Adult Family Members' Orientation for Intensive Care Units

I. Introduction

II. Purpose of unit

    A. Number of beds

    B. Patient populations

III. Health care professionals and roles of each

    A. Critical care nurses

    B. Physicians

    C. Respiratory therapists

    D. Unit clerks

    E. Dieticians

    F. Pharmacists

    G. Others

IV. Communication

    A. Importance

    B. Ways to communicate

    C. A spokesperson

V. Visiting

    A. Options

    B. Access to the patient

    C. Lounge

    D. Taking care of yourself

VI. Infection control and safety

    A. Health of visitors

    B. Hand washing

    C. Special considerations

VII. The critical care environment

    A. Description of equipment

    B. Noises

    C. Patient's response/reaction to the environment

    D. Family role

VIII. Resources available to families

Source: Used with permission by the Family Intervention Research Team, University of Iowa Hospitals and Clinics and The University of Iowa College of Nursing, Iowa City, Iowa.

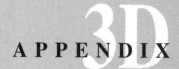
Sample Intervention Checklist for the First Visit of an Adult Family Member to a Critically Ill Adult Patient

Date: _____

❏ Introduce self to each family member.

❏ Ask/confirm relationship of family member to the patient.

❏ Ask if the family member has been in a CCU before.

❏ Ask about the family member's condition. (How are you doing? Are you getting any sleep? Do you have a place to stay tonight?)

   ❏ Explain, in understandable terms, the reasons for the patient being in the ICU.

   ❏ Describe the patient's bedside environment, the equipment present, and the appearance and psychosocial behavior of the patient. ("Your mother has a tube in her airway helping her to breathe so she cannot talk to you but she can nod yes or no.")

   ❏ Describe the physiological stability of the patient, in understandable terms.

   ❏ Describe to family members the sights and sounds associated with a CCU.

   ❏ Instruct family members on actions to take for infection control and safety.

❏ Wash hands on entering and leaving the unit or room.

❏ Refrain from visiting if you have symptoms of a communicable disease (sore throat, cold, fever) or if you have been diagnosed with a communicable disease (eg, strep throat).

❏ Refrain from moving equipment; call the nurse if you have questions.

❏ Call the nurse if you (the family member) start feeling lightheaded or feel you are going to faint. You can also sit down, or go back to the waiting area, escorted by another family member.

   ❏ Give family members written information about the unit and review it with them (this should include ICU visiting guidelines and critical care instruction book).

   ❏ Instruct and review specific steps to take with each visit.

   ❏ Provide an opportunity for family to ask questions before and following the visit.

   ❏ Inform family that they may be asked to leave the unit in certain situations such as emergencies or when certain procedures are performed.

   ❏ Encourage family on positive interactions with the patient (eg, holding hand, communicating in an appropriate manner).

Signature of person completing the form: _____

Source: Used with permission by the Family Intervention Research Team, University of Iowa Hospitals and Clinics and The University of Iowa College of Nursing, Iowa City, Iowa.

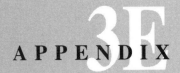
Child Visitation in Adult and Neonatal Critical Care Units

Age Group	Developmental Task	Typical Behaviors of Age Group	Interventions

3-5 years	Initiative vs guilt	Some separation anxiety (crying)
		
		Fear of abandonment, mutilation, loss of parental love
		
		Views illness as punishment
		
		Guilt
		
		Dependence-independence conflicts
		
		With stress may witness:
		• Increased fears and crying
		• Regression
		• Withdrawal
		• Acting out
			• Set realistic limits on behavior.
			• Allow for expression of emotions.
			• Reassure child he or she is not at fault.
			
			Before the visit:
			• Provide clear, simple explanations.
			• Refer to body parts using photos.
			• Use visual, auditory, tactile means (dolls, puppets, art) to provide explanations.
			• Use concrete terms.
			
			After the visit:
			• Use pictures or toys to initiate dialogue.
			• Have child color or draw picture and use as focus of discussion. (Note important cues such as omission of self; position and size of family members.)
			• Ask simple questions:
			  • "Tell me about your visit."
			  • "Do you have questions?"
			• Allow expression of emotions.

Age Group	Developmental Task	Typical Behaviors of Age Group	Interventions
5-10 years	Industry vs inferiority	More stable, conceptual organization of thinking Invested in nonfamily members May experience disillusionment with parents	*Before the visit:* • Prepare for the sights and sounds of the unit by describing machinery, tubes; use simple but direct language. • Assure the child that the staff have cared for patients with the same disease many times. • Assure the child that equipment is being used only to help the patient and will be removed as soon as the patient no longer needs it. • Tell the child that many people feel overwhelmed by the experience of visiting intensive care, and that he or she can ask to leave at any time without risk of embarrassment. • Forewarn the child that adults have feelings too and may cry. • Show child what he or she can do at the bedside. *After the visit:* • Clarify information. • Reaffirm feelings. • Review some ways to help relieve stress (eg, talking with others, imagery).
11-17 years	Establishing identity	Conflict between family beliefs and pressures of peers and society Parents often discredited Loosens family ties Work and responsibility habits solidify Moody, uncommunicative with family members Importance of conformity to peer group Wishes for independence Substance abuse common	*Before the visit:* • Prepare for sights and sounds of ICU. • Give explanations in as much detail as the young person requests. • Explain that many adults are overwhelmed at visiting the ICU, and that he or she may ask to leave at any time without embarrassment. *After the visit:* • Validate feelings. • Reaffirm the adolescent's own needs. • Stress the importance of open communication between family members during ties of crisis. • Stress the importance of maintaining peer relationships during times of crisis. • Review possible coping strategies. • Emphasize the importance of avoiding substance abuse.

Source: Used with permission by the Family Intervention Research Team, University of Iowa Hospitals and Clinics and The University of Iowa College of Nursing, Iowa City, Iowa.

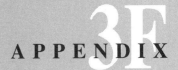
Sample Form for Health Screening for Communicable Diseases for Use with Child Visits in Critical Care

Before visiting in the special care nursery or adult ICU, visitors under 14 years of age must be screened for the following conditions. Any child with a positive history or assessment of disease may be restricted from visiting at this time (see Appendix G for guidelines).

Patient being visited: _____

Visitor's name: _____

Has the visitor been exposed to or had any of the following within the past 4 weeks?

❏ Chicken pox/shingles   ❏ Roseola

❏ Mumps   ❏ Fifth disease (parvovirus)

❏ German measles (rubella)   ❏ Tuberculosis

❏ Croup   ❏ Respiratory syncytial virus

❏ Strep throat (last 7 days)   ❏ Hepatitis

❏ Measles (rubeola)

Does the visitor have any of the following?

❏ Sore throat   ❏ Open wound or sore

❏ Rash   ❏ Gastroenteritis/diarrhea

❏ Cold sore/herpes infection   ❏ Upper respiratory illness/runny nose

❏ Fever   ❏ Conjunctivitis, red eyes

❏ Cough

❏ Has the visitor received polio immunization within the past 4 weeks?

❏ Has the visitor received the chicken pox vaccine within the past 4 weeks?

Source: Used with permission by the Family Intervention Research Team, University of Iowa Hospitals and Clinics and The University of Iowa College of Nursing, Iowa City, Iowa.

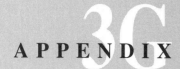
Guidelines for Action with a Positive Finding on the Health Screening Form for Use with Child Visits in Critical Care

I. Exposure is defined as being in the same room, either interacting together or being side by side, with someone who has the disease or breaks out with the disease within 24 hours after the contact.

II. Types of exposure and actions

A. *Chicken pox/shingles:* The incubation period of chicken pox is up to 28 days. The person who has been exposed is considered contagious during 7 to 28 days after exposure and thus should not visit during this period of time. The visitor who has been exposed to this virus and has already had chicken pox is not at risk of developing chicken pox and, therefore, is not a risk to the patient.

B. *Measles, mumps, German measles (rubella) (MMR):* Visitors who have had the MMR immunization and are asymptomatic are not at risk, and they may visit. Visitors who have not had the immunization may not visit during the incubation period.

Incubation periods

• German measles: 12 to 23 days after exposure

• Measles: 7 to 18 days after exposure

• Mumps: 12 to 25 days after exposure

C. *Roseola:* Visitors may not visit during the incubation period (5-15 days after exposure).

D. *Strep throat:* Visitors who have been exposed to a known case of strep throat in the past 5 to 7 days should not visit even if the visitor has not developed signs or symptoms of the disease.

E. *Pneumonia:* Visitors who have symptoms may not visit. Those who are asymptomatic may visit despite exposure to pneumonia.

F. *Hepatitis:* Because of the multiple types of hepatitis, as well as the varying incubation and shedding periods, any visitor who has been exposed to hepatitis should not visit until hospital epidemiology and infection control personnel are contacted and permission is granted.

G. *Fifth disease (Erythema infectiosum):* Visitors may not visit during the incubation period (4-20 days after exposure).

H. *Respiratory syncytial virus (RSV):* Visitors may not visit during the incubation period (2-8 days after exposure).

I. *Croup:* Visitors may not visit during the incubation period (1-10 days after exposure).

J. *Tuberculosis:* Visitors with prolonged, close contact to a person with pulmonary or laryngeal tuberculosis should not visit. Visitors with any kind of therapy for tuberculosis should not visit until hospital epidemiology and infection control personnel are contacted, evaluate the specific case, and grant permission to visit.

K. *Polio:* Visitors who have received a polio immunization in the past 6 weeks should not visit, especially immunocompromised patients, because people can shed the virus for up to 6 weeks.

III. Symptoms. The following are guidelines for positive symptom screen:

1. *Sore throat, fever, gastroenteritis, diarrhea:* Visitors should not visit an adult patient.

2. *Upper respiratory illness, cough, runny nose:* Visitors should wear a mask when in the patient area. Some visitors may not visit an adult inpatient based on the patients illness (eg, immunosuppressed). Visitors should not visit if fever is present.

3. *Cold sore or herpes infection:* Visitors should not visit an immunocompromised adult patient and must wear a mask to visit a nonimmunocompromised patient.

4. *Open wound or sore:* Must be covered with dry dressing. If there is any question, hospital epidemiology or infection control should be consulted to make the final decision.

5. *Rash:* Visitors should not visit if a rash is present unless it is a known contact dermatitis or allergic reaction.

6. *Red eyes, conjunctivitis:* Visitors should not visit unless it is a known allergic reaction or other known condition that is noncontagious.

IV. Hospital epidemiology or infection control personnel can be contacted to clarify guidelines, report exposures, or facilitate decision making about a child's health and potential exposure to the patient.

Reinforce the need for hand washing on entering and leaving the patient's room.

Source: Used with permission by the Family Intervention Research Team, University of Iowa Hospitals and Clinics and the University of Iowa College of Nursing, Iowa City, Iowa.

Family Pet Visiting and Animal-Assisted Therapy

Nancy C. Molter, RN, MN, PhD

Family Pet Visiting and Animal-Assisted Therapy

CASE STUDY

Mr G had been in the medical ICU for 33 long, painful, frightening, and frustrating days. Mr G had a life-long history of hospital visits related to complications from childhood polio. Severe curvature of the spine caused restrictive lung disease problems, and the deformity of his legs forced him to get around at home on a little scooter. A cold had turned into pneumonia, which precipitated septic shock, which led to renal insufficiency. Just when it looked as if Mr G was going to pull through this severe assault on his fragile body, many other complications intervened to prolong his hospital stay. Maintaining Mr G's fluid balance was like walking a tightrope: Just a little bit one way or the other led to a decrease in oxygenation, hypotension, or tachycardia. Mr G was unable to avoid complications of gastrointestinal bleeding and another bout with pneumonia before he succeeded in being weaned from the ventilator. But then a second bout with a bleeding ulcer put him back on the ventilator after he had been off for 48 hours.

Mr G was one of those rare people who goes through a lifetime of difficult challenges while retaining an attitude and personality that everyone adored. Many neighbors and friends visited. His wife read to him, gave him back rubs, did his bath, tried to do as much as she could of his care, and was by his side most of the day. It was easy for a nurse to care for Mr G. He always mouthed "please" and "thank you" for any little thing you did. He always tried his very best to do what you asked, whether it was using the incentive spirometer, holding very still for central line placements and feeding tubes, or doing exercises for physical therapy. And we called on all the therapies we had: music therapy, physical therapy, relaxation therapy, and a daily schedule

that strategically mapped out times for weaning trials, rest, exercise, and bath.

However, Mr G's hospital course was more than any person could cope with. He began having anxiety spells and days of feeling depressed and hopeless, especially when another complication affected his progress. So began a cycle of anxiety-lorazepam-sleep-anxiety, depression-lorazepam-sleep, and so on.

Mr G's wife was the one to suggest a therapy we hadn't used—a therapy that didn't require any effort on the patient's part, didn't hurt, didn't beep or poke. It did, however, wiggle with ecstasy when it saw Mr G. An orange bundle of fur named Pumpkin did more to alleviate Mr G's anxiety and depression than any drug or therapy. Pumpkin provided a dose of something that isn't easily measured. The visit of Mr G's beloved dog didn't cure his illnesses, but it did make him smile, relax, and reminisce.

Mr G left the medical ICU a week later. Whether the pet visiting had anything to do with that is hard to measure. However, animals are proving to be an excellent intervention that nurses can use to give the best of care and help meet the patient's needs.

GENERAL DESCRIPTION

Pets are often viewed as family members and were included in the definition of family by the members of the consensus conference on fostering more humane critical care (Other References: 11). Animal visiting programs vary from having patients' pets visit them in the hospital to programs that have set criteria for training animals and their owners for use in animal-assisted activities and animal-assisted therapy. The benefits of pet or animal visiting include decreased feelings of loneliness, increased socialization, and decreases in physiological indices such as heart rate (HR), blood pressure (BP), and respiratory rate (RR). Pet or animal visiting in long-term care settings has been in use for several years. More recently there has been increased interest in pets visiting in acute and ICUs. Most pet visiting concentrates on facilitating interactions between a patient and a dog, but cats and rabbits also come into play (Annotated Bibliography: 3, 4; Suggested Readings: 4).

Two types of programs are usually considered. In the first type, an animal and owner undergo training for visiting in a health care setting through programs such as the Delta Society Pet Partners Program (Suggested Readings: 8). The animal-owner team undergoes a behavior screen that focuses on the behavior of the animal in various situations, and the owner provides evidence of a recent animal health screen. This is usually referred to as *animal-assisted therapy* (AAT), a therapeutic approach of bringing animals and people with physical or emotional needs together for a specified goal and as an integral part of treatment (Suggested Readings: 8). With *animal-assisted activities* (AAA), also carried out by a certified animal-owner team, the activity is repeated with different people, unlike a therapy program that is tailored for a particular patient to achieve an identified goal over time (Suggested Readings: 10, 14-16).

In the second type of program, family pet visiting, there is facilitated interaction between a patient and that patient's own pet. The pet is bathed no more than 24 hours before the visit, a health screen is completed, evidence of updated immunizations for the pet are provided, and arrangements are made for the pet to visit the family member (Other References: 4).

Pet visiting and AAA or AAT are generally used for patients who like animals and are neither allergic to animals nor immunosuppressed. Proper administration of these programs will minimize any possible associated hazards such as bites, scratches, or infections transmitted from animals to humans. Anyone interested in using this intervention is encouraged to work with the institution's administration and infection control personnel to ensure appropriate policies and procedures are in place to carry out this intervention safely and effectively.

Benefits

The lulling, rhythmic, repetitive nature of petting a companion dog is a passive, meditative focus on a nonthreatening stimulus that has the potential to relax a person by lowering his or her state of arousal. Studies have shown that petting a companion dog decreases BP in healthy subjects, and decreases BP and increases peripheral skin temperature in hypertensive subjects (Annotated Bibliography: 1, 2, 5; Other References: 3; Suggested Readings: 2, 7). Other investigators using subjects with hypertension have demonstrated that blood pressure decreased over time when petting a familiar dog and an unknown dog, and peripheral skin temperatures increased more (indicating relaxation) when petting a com-

panion dog than when petting an unknown dog (Other References: 7, 8). Studies suggest that in the long-term, interacting with pets results in decreased risk for cardiovascular disease, morbidity, and mortality (Annotated Bibliography: 1, 4, 6; Suggested Readings: 7, 15).

Studies have focused on the psychosocial and emotional benefits of pet visiting (Other References: 1, 5, 12, 13; Suggested Readings: 7, 14). Psychological benefits are improved self-esteem, greater feelings of security (Other References: 4), reduced stress and anxiety (Other References: 9, 10), decreased loneliness (Annotated Bibliography: 3), improved social interaction, communication (Annotated Bibliography: 6; Other References: 1), and sensory stimulation (Annotated Bibliography: 4). These studies suggest that people experiencing stress, either acutely or chronically, may benefit from short-term interactions with their pet that serve to focus attention away from the stressor and to a more pleasurable, calming interaction. Most of these studies, however, have been done with chronic mentally ill and geriatric patients, or with acute psychiatric inpatients. The benefit of pet visiting or AAA or AAT in critical care is mainly anecdotal; there are few randomized, controlled trials with critically ill patients (Suggested Readings: 7).

COMPETENCY

Competency requirements vary depending on which type of program is implemented. The two common types of programs are family pet visiting and certified animal-owner teams (AAA or AAT).

Family Pet Visiting

Many patients who consider the family pet as a member of the family unit may request a visit from their beloved pet. Some institutions do not provide guidance to meet such requests, with the result that pets are smuggled into patients' rooms. The following guidelines can be used to assist in permitting pets to visit (guidelines vary by institution):

1. The person who plans to bring in the pet should discuss with the nurse manager (or designee) the best time to visit and the best route to reach the patient's room or designated visit area. Use designated elevators, stairways, and halls in consideration of those with allergies.
2. The attending physician may need to write an order for the pet to visit (follow institutional guidelines) after allergy implications for the patient have been addressed.
3. Pets other than dogs or cats should be cleared through a veterinarian or the hospital epidemiologist. A pet visit program health certificate should be completed for all pets (Appendix 4-A).
4. A pet should be bathed no more than 24 hours before the visit and be free from fleas.
5. A designated professional will assess the pet before the visit for cleanliness; absence of fleas, sores, or open

areas on the skin; and to ensure that the pet has been feeling well (no diarrhea or vomiting). All vaccinations should be current with a confirmatory signed certificate from the veterinarian. If there is any doubt about any of these assessments, the visit should be canceled.

6. All involved should wash their hands before and after handling the pet.

7. A designated area for visiting should be agreed on. If the visit is planned for a patient in a double room, then the roommate should agree to the pet visit and be free from designated animal allergies.

8. A sheet should be placed over the bed before the patient handles the pet or the pet is allowed to be on the bed.

9. A pet visiting sign should be placed on the door to indicate a visit is in progress.

10. The pet should be on a leash at all times and under control of the person responsible for bringing it to the facility.

11. The pet is the responsibility of the person who brought it into the hospital and who should remain with the pet during the visit.

12. The person bringing the pet to the hospital should be prepared to clean up and dispose of pet excrement properly (Other References: 4).

See Appendix 4-A for samples of family pet visiting forms.

Animal-Assisted Activities and Animal-Assisted Therapy

Both AAA and AAT involve a certified or screened animal-owner team visiting patients. Certified animal-owner teams usually consist of a volunteer with pet (eg, dog, cat) that has been certified to visit in a health care setting. The certification indicates that the animal has passed a series of health screening and behavioral tests that confer some degree of competency to visit patients on the part of the team. The Delta Society, which distinguishes between AAA and AAT (Table 4-1), has standards and a certification program for animal-owner teams (Suggested Readings: 7, 8, 10, 14, 15). See Appendix B for information on how to contact the Delta Society, an organization devoted to the enhancement of the human-animal bond, which is the most comprehensive source of materials on the subject of AAA and AAT.

General

Proper administrative channels must have been used in order to institute family pet visiting, AAA, or AAT. Initial development and implementation of such programs are best done by a multidisciplinary team that includes someone from infection control or hospital epidemiology (Annotated Bibliography: 4; Suggested Readings: 5, 9, 12, 13; Other References: 6). Patient inclusion and exclusion criteria for participating in family pet visiting and AAA or AAT programs help in making decisions about whether to use this intervention for a specific patient (Annotated Bibliography: 3; Other References: 4; Suggested Readings: 10, 13, 15).

ETHICAL CONSIDERATIONS

Pet visiting by the patient's pet or by a trained certified dog-owner team has for years been affected by the pervasive mind-set that dogs, cats, and other pets are dirty, uncontrollable, unpredictable, and disease-ridden pests. But when you consider that 54% of households in the United States own a pet, and many of these people eat, sleep, and travel with their pet, it is clear a wide range of beliefs prevails in our society. It is extremely important not to interfere with a person's right to chose if he or she wants to be exposed to animals (Suggested Readings: 9). Policies and procedures should ensure that family pet visiting does not interfere with these rights. Dossey suggests that the "Evidence favoring the health value of pets is so compelling that if pet therapy were a pill, we would not be able to manufacture it fast enough" (Suggested Readings: 7, p. 15).

COMPLICATIONS

Possible hazards associated with family pet visiting and AAA or AAT are bites, scratches, and zoonotic infections (infections that can be passed from animal to human). Most

Table 4-1 Animal-Assisted Activities and Animal-Assisted Therapy	
Animal-Assisted Activities (AAA)	**Animal-Assisted Therapy (AAT)**
• The animal-owner team visits people for motivational, educational, or recreational benefits to enhance the quality of life, and the visit or activity is repeated with different people. • Specially trained professionals, paraprofessionals, or volunteers in association with animals that meet specific criteria deliver AAA in a variety of environments.	• The visit is tailored to a particular person or people with a similar medical condition. • In this goal-directed intervention, an animal that meets specific criteria is an integral part of the treatment process. • The professional identifies specific goals for each client, and measures and records progress. • AAT is designed to promote improvement in physical, social, emotional, or cognitive functioning.

Source: Delta Society (Suggested Readings: 10).

possible transmissions are prevented by good hand washing. The use of certified screened animals is one way to prevent infections, bites, or injury from a frightened animal that is not used to the hospital setting (Suggested Readings: 10). Screened AAA or AAT animals are tested to see how they react to pain, loud noises, equipment, and strange human behavior. Schantz (Suggested Readings: 9), Weber and colleagues (Suggested Readings: 12), and Brodie et al. (Suggested Readings 13) discuss in detail zoonotic infections of potential concern when using pets and animals in institutions. The Pet Assisted Therapy program at Huntington Memorial Hospital in Pasadena, California, reports that in 8000 visits to 6000 patients they have never experienced an episode of zoonotic infection. General principles to consider when formulating a policy for the use of pets in institutions include the need to perform the following:

- Select the animal carefully to keep the threat of an animal bite to a minimum.
- Avoid exposure of animal-allergic patients to animals.
- Implement a comprehensive infection control program for family pets and other animals.
- Formulate family pet visiting and AAA or AAT policies with advice from public health veterinarians, physicians, administrators, and infection control officers.
- Develop plans for surveillance and response to emergency situations. (Suggested Readings: 9).

FUTURE RESEARCH

Family pet visiting and AAA or AAT need further research. Much of the research to date has been done with small samples, and the majority has focused on the elderly, mentally ill, or healthy subjects. Little research has been done on animal visits in the critical care setting, and there is little empirical evidence to refute or support family pet visiting and AAA or AAT with critically ill patients. Many articles can be found on anecdotal situations where a patient shows great benefit from an animal visit. Randomized controlled trials are needed to explicate the potential short- and long-term benefits of family pet visiting and AAA or AAT in critical care.

Methodological barriers such as gaining access to clinical sites, overcoming organizational resistance to allowing animals to be with immunocompromised patients, recruiting ethnic and age-diverse populations, and randomization and sample size issues must be addressed with creativity and good research design (Suggested Readings: 17). In the acute and critical care environment, research might focus on the effects of assisted-animal therapy on ventilatory weaning, pain medication requirements, length of stay, body image, functional improvement measures and patient education retention (Suggested Readings: 14).

SUGGESTED READINGS

1. Barba B. The positive influence of animals: AAT in acute care. *Clin Nurse Specialist.* 1995;9(4):199-202.
2. Baun MM, Oetting K, Bergstrom N. Health benefits of companion animals in relation to the physiologic indices of relaxation. *Holistic Nurs Pract.* 1991; 5(2):16-23.
3. Bernard S. *Animal Assisted Therapy—A Guide for Health Care Professionals and Volunteers.* Whitehouse, Tex: Therapet LLC; 1995.
4. Brickel CM. Pet-facilitated therapies. A review of the literature and clinical implementation considerations. *Clin Gerontologist.* 1986;5:309-331.
5. Carmack B, Fila D. Animal-assisted therapy: a nursing intervention. *Nurs Manage.* 1989;20(5):96,98,100-101.
6. Davis JH. Animal-facilitated therapy. *Holistic Nurs Pract.* 1988;2(3):75-83.
7. Dossey, L. The healing power of pets: a look at animal-assisted therapy. *Alternative Ther.* 1997;3(4):8-16.
8. Fredrickson M. *Pet Partners Program. Introductory Handler Skills Course for Animal-Assisted Activities and Therapy. Home Study Version.* 2nd ed. Renton, Wash: Delta Society; 1996.
9. Schantz P. Preventing potential health hazards incidental to the use of pets in therapy. *Anthrozoos.* 1990; 4(1):14-23.
10. *Standards of Practice for Animal-Assisted Activities and Therapy.* Renton, Wash: Delta Society; 1996:1-92.
11. Waltner-Toews D, Ellis A. *Good for Your Animals, Good for You: How to Live and Work With Animals in Activity and Therapy Programs and Stay Healthy.* Guelph, Canada: The University of Guelph; 1994.
12. Weber DJ, Baker AS, Rutala WA. Epidemiology and prevention of nosocomial infections associated with animals in the hospital. In: MayHall BG, ed. *Hospital Epidemiology and Infection Control.* Baltimore, Md: Williams & Wilkins; 1996:1109-1125.
13. Brodie SJ, Biley FC, Shewring M. An exploration of the potential risks associated with using pet therapy in healthcare settings. *J Clin Nurs.* 2002;11:444-456.
14. Connor C, Miller J. Animal-assisted therapy: an in-depth look. *Dimens Crit Care Nurs.* 2000;19(3):20-26.
15. Fine AH, ed. *Handbook of Animal Assisted Therapy: Theoretical Foundations and Guidelines for Practice.* San Diego, Calif: The Academic Press; 1999.
16. Giuliano KK, Bloniasz E, Bell J. Implementation of a pet visitation program in critical care. *Crit Care Nurs.* 1999;19(3):43-50.
17. Johnson RA, Odendaal JSJ, Meadows RL. Animal-assisted interventions research: issues and answers. *West J Nurs Res.* 2002;24(4):422-440.

CLINICAL RECOMMENDATIONS

The rating scale for the Level of Recommendation ranges from I to VI, with levels indicated as follows: I, manufacturer's recommendations only; II, theory based, no research data to support recommendations; recommendations from expert consensus group may exist; III, laboratory data only, no clinical data to support recommendations; IV, limited clinical studies to support recommendations; V, clinical studies in more than 1 or 2 different populations and situations to support recommendations; VI, clinical studies in a variety of patient populations and situations to support recommendations.

Period of Use	Recommendation	Rationale for Recommendation	Level of Recommendation	Supporting References	Comments
Selection of Patients	Adult and pediatric patients who are not immunocompromised and have no • Known animal allergies • Fear of animals	Animal visits may trigger an allergic response. Visits by the family pet or an animal should be by the patient's choice and a pleasant experience.	IV: Limited clinical studies to support recommendations	See Suggested Readings: 1, 4, 9, 11, 12, 13	Family pet visiting, AAA, and AAT are controversial for the immunocompromised patient. Special consideration may be warranted for patients who are unpredictable or violent, as they may hurt or provoke animals. Appendix B lists resources for AAA and AAT.
	• Splenectomy	Patients who have a splenectomy have a heightened susceptibility to digenic fermenter types (DF2), a gram-negative bacterium that is among the normal flora in dog saliva.			
	• Isolation precautions				
Application and Initial Use	*Patient Assessment* Ask the patient the following questions: • Have you ever owned a pet? • What type of pets have you owned? • Do you own a pet now? • Are you afraid of dogs? cats? • Do you have allergies to dogs? cats? other animals? • What is your pet's name? • How would you describe your pet: a companion? best friend? • Would you like an animal (eg, dog, cat, other animal) or your pet to visit?	A comprehensive assessment of the patient's perception of companion animals provides a basis for considering family pet visiting and AAA or AAT as a stress mediator.	II: Theory based, no research data to support recommendations; recommendations from expert consensus group may exist	See Suggested Readings: 1, 3, 5, 6, 14, 15, 16	The type of visit (family pet visiting, AAA or AAT) offered depends on the program offered in the organization.

Period of Use	Recommendation	Rationale for Recommendation	Level of Recommendation	Supporting References	Comments
Application and Initial Use (*cont.*)	*Plan for Family Pet Visiting, AAA, or AAT*				
	Instruct owner or person bringing the pet or animal to the hospital of the hospital protocol, such as need for:	Pet owner is responsible for behavior of pet.	IV: Limited clinical studies to support recommendations	See Suggested Readings: 5, 6, 9, 12, 13, 15	Agencies instituting AAA or AAT should refer to Delta Society information (Appendix B).
	• Signed health screening form				
	• Temperament screen				
	• Bathing within 24 hours of visit				
	• Entrance and route to the unit				
	• Time of planned visit				
	• Animal on leash at all times				
	• How to handle animal excrement				
	Family Pet Assessment				
	Obtain veterinary certification of family pet's health.	Assessment avoids chance of unnecessarily exposing the patient to potential harm.	IV: Limited clinical studies to support recommendations	See Suggested Readings: 3, 6, 9, 14, 16	
	Review family pet temperament with person bringing pet to the hospital.				
	Examine family pet for cleanliness and freedom from fleas, ticks, open wounds, or sores.				
	For AAA or AAT, contact the Delta Society.			See Suggested Readings: 7, 9	See resource list in Appendix B.
	Facilitate Family Pet or Animal and Patient Interaction				
	Instruct all to wash hands before visit.	Decreases chance of contaminating area and alerts others to presence of an animal	IV: Limited clinical studies to support recommendations	See Annotated Bibliography: 3	
	Ask patient where pet or animal should sit (eg, floor, bed).			See Suggested Readings: 1, 3, 4, 5, 7, 12, 14, 16, 17	
	Place sheet over patient to serve as a barrier.			See Other References: 6,	
	Place "pet visit in progress" sign on door.				

Period of Use	Recommendation	Rationale for Recommendation	Level of Recommendation	Supporting References	Comments
Ongoing Monitoring	*Patient and Pet or Animal*				
	Monitor patient's HR, BP, RR.	HR, BP may initially increase and then decline.	IV: Limited clinical studies to support recommendations	See Annotated Bibliography: 2, 3, 5, 6 See Other References: 3 See Suggested Readings: 1, 2, 4, 6, 14, 16	Contact the Delta Society for detailed information on AAA and AAT (Appendix B).
	Observe patient's affect and behavioral response (smile, communication).	Positive behaviors of patient indicate positive interaction with animal.			
	Monitor the animal's response to people and the environment.	If family pet or animal becomes anxious or restless, the visit may need to be terminated. Length of visit should be gauged by energy level of the patient and stamina of the animal.		See Other References: 6 See Suggested Readings: 7, 10, 14, 16	
	Instruct all to wash hands at completion of visit.				
	Program Evaluation				
	Type of family pets and animals used for AAA or AAT Number of visits Demographics of patients participating	Systematic evaluation is needed to: • Measure achievement of program goals • Keep program documents updated and in order • Refine the program to meet patient needs	IV: Limited clinical studies to support recommendations	See Annotated Bibliography: 3 See Suggested Readings: 1, 16	
	Adequacy of physical facilities: • Route to unit • Visitation space Incident reports Patient satisfaction Positive and negative experiences				
Prevention of Complications	Reinforce hospital policy to all areas participating in family pet visiting and AAA or AAT program. Review hospital policy yearly. Agree, as an institution, the types of patients to include and exclude from family pet visiting and AAA or AAT.	Minimizes risk of complications		See Other References: 3 See Suggested Readings: 1, 9, 12, 14, 16	For a safe, successful program, a governing body is recommended to reinforce compliance to policies and procedures.

Period of Use	Recommendation	Rationale for Recommendation	Level of Recommendation	Supporting References	Comments
Prevention of Complications *(cont.)*	Implement a comprehensive infection control program for family pets and animals used for AAA and AAT.				For more information on infection control contact the Association for Practitioners in Infection Control (APIC), 1016 16th Street NW, 6th Floor, Washington, DC 20036 (202) 296-2742.
	Develop a plan for surveillance and response to emergency situations.	Staff should know how to act in case of an adverse occurrence.			
Quality Control Issues	Assure health screening of animals is completed. Inspect animals for cleanliness, etc., before each visit.	To decrease risk of infection	IV: Limited clinical studies to support recommendations	See Annotated Bibliography: 3 See Other References: 3, 6, See Suggested Readings: 9, 12, 13, 14, 16	Some institutions may require a physician's order for family pet visiting and AAA or AAT.
	Assess patient for contraindications to family pet visiting and AAA or AAT.	To prevent allergic reactions, infection			

ANNOTATED BIBLIOGRAPHY

1. Anderson WP, Reid CM, Jennings GL. Pet ownership and risk factors for cardiovascular disease. *Med J Aust.* 1992;157:298-301.

Study Sample

Subjects for this study were 5741 adults (3394 men and 2347 women), ages 20 to 60 years, who were self-referred to the Baker Medical Research Institute's Cardiovascular Disease Risk Evaluation Clinic at Monash University Medical School in Melbourne, Australia. The subjects, recruited to be representative of the Australian population, had a cardiovascular risk profile very similar to that of the National Heart Foundation of Australia.

Comparison Studied

The purpose of the study was to determine any association of pet ownership with reduced levels of identified cardiovascular risk factors.

Study Procedures

On arriving at the clinic, and after giving informed consent, participants completed a lifestyle questionnaire relating to smoking habits and personal and family history of heart disease. Two supine blood pressure measurements were taken after 5 and 10 minutes of rest, then venous blood was drawn to measure cholesterol and triglycerides. Subjects who owned a pet completed a brief questionnaire about pets. Blood pressure, plasma cholesterol, and triglyceride levels were compared between 784 pet owners and 4957 subjects who didn't own pets.

Key Results

Pet owners had significantly lower systolic blood pressure and plasma triglycerides than nonowners. There were no differences in body mass indices and smoking habits were similar, but pet owners reported that they exercised more than nonowners and ate more meat and take-out foods. The socioeconomic profiles of the pet owners and nonowners were comparable.

Study Strengths and Weaknesses

The lower risk factor of individual pet owners could have been confounded by other unmeasured cardiovascular risk factors. A prospective, controlled trial is needed to confirm the findings of this cross-sectional study. The large sample size and keeping subjects blinded to asking about pet ownership until physiological data were collected are strengths of this study.

Clinical Implications

This study suggests that owning a pet reduces cardiovascular risk factors that could not be explained by cigarette smoking, diet, body mass, or socioeconomic status.

2. Baun MM, Bergstrom N, Langston NF, Thomas L. Physiological effects of human/companion animal bonding. *Nurs Res.* 1984;33:126-129.

Study Sample

Twenty-four healthy subjects (5 men and 19 women), 24 to 74 years of age, formed the study sample. Subjects were free from hypertension; were not taking medication known to affect BP, HR, or RR; were not allergic to dogs; and had a dog with whom they had established some degree of bonding.

Comparison Studied

The authors sought to determine in three 9-minute sessions (reading quietly, petting one's own dog, and petting a strange dog) if there was a difference in the physiological reactions of people to petting dogs when a companion bond had been or had not been established. Subjects served as their own controls and the order of the intervention was random.

Study Procedures

Blood pressure was measured electronically; HR was measured via a three-electrode ECG monitor; RR was measured using a Thermister respiration transducer placed in the nostril in the subject's nondominant side. Subjects sat quietly for 10 minutes with the measurement devices in place before being exposed to the three treatments. Blood pressure, HR, and RR were measured at baseline and at 3-minute intervals during each of the 9-minute sessions.

Key Results

Petting a companion dog resulted in a significantly greater decline in systolic and diastolic BP compared to petting an unknown dog. This decline paralleled the relaxing effects of reading. Other results showed a "greeting response" to the entry of a dog with whom the subject had a bond, which resulted in an initial increase in BP higher than the response to the unknown dog and to reading. Respiratory rate declined over time but there were nonsignificant differences in responses from the companion dog and the unknown dog.

Study Strengths and Weaknesses

This is a well-designed study with little threat to internal or external validity. This study should be replicated using subjects with acute or chronic illness.

Clinical Implications

This study suggests a positive hemodynamic response in healthy subjects to interaction with a companion pet.

3. Cole KM, Gawlinski A. Animal-assisted therapy in the intensive care unit. A staff nurse's dream comes true. *Nurs Clin North Am.* 1995;30: 529-537.

Study Sample

Subjects were those wishing to interact with a dog while being cared for in the coronary or intermediate care units at the UCLA Medical Center over a 6-month period.

Comparison Studied

In this program evaluation study, research findings were used to change practice to permit visitation by a trained volunteer handler or dog team.

Study Procedures

Trained volunteer handler or dog teams made 120 visits to patients' rooms. Each patient was given a questionnaire following the visit that assessed 8 positive and 8 negative affective adjectives. A planned change approach was used to institute this practice.

Key Results

The patients indicated unanimously that the visits made them either calmer, happier, or less lonely. Half the patients also indicated that a program like this would affect their choice of hospital. All said they would recommend this program to a friend or relative.

Study Strengths and Weaknesses

This is an excellent example of a research-based change in practice with a strong evaluation component.

Clinical Implications

An animal visiting program can be successfully implemented in a coronary and intermediate care unit using research and planned change to implement the practice.

4. Friedman E, Katcher A, Lynch J, Thomas SA. Animal companions and one-year survival of patients after discharge from a coronary care unit. *Public Health Rep.* 1980;95:307-312.

Study Sample

Ninety-six white patients (29 women and 67 men), ages 37 to 79, with a diagnosis of myocardial infarction or angina pectoris were invited to participate in this study from August 1975 to March 1977.

Comparison Studied

The purpose of this study was to examine the effect of social isolation and social support on survival of patients hospitalized in a cardiac care unit. Specifically, the association between pet ownership and survival were examined.

Study Procedures

Subjects, who were interviewed in the hospital, completed an inventory of social data and an adjective checklist for psychological mood status. Pet ownership was also assessed.

A modified coronary prognostic index was used to describe physiologic severity of each subject. All surviving patients were contacted after 1 year.

Key Results

In the cohort of 92 subjects available at 1 year, 53 (58%) had 1 or more pets at 1 year, and 78 (84%) were still alive at 1 year. Of the 39 patients who did not have pets, 11 (28%) had died whereas only 3 (6%) of the pet owners had died. Pet ownership was correlated with survival but not with physiological severity. The relationship of pet ownership to survival was similar for men and women.

Study Strengths and Weaknesses

The major limitation is the unexplained association between pet ownership and 1-year survival. Those who have pets may be more physically active because of the care requirements of the pet, which in turn would have a positive impact on cardiac outcomes. This study provides empirical data for future studies regarding pet ownership and cardiac survival.

Clinical Implications

The therapeutic use of pets should be considered for patients with coronary heart disease, and the existence of pets as important household members should be considered by those responsible for medical treatment.

5. Vormbrock J, Grossberg JM. Cardiovascular effects of human-pet dog interactions. *J Behav Med.* 1988;11:509-517.

Study Sample

Subjects were 30 male and 30 female undergraduates, 18 to 24 years of age, with normal BP. Subjects were selected from a pool of 461 students based on scores on the Pet Attitude Scale and their Liking for Pet Dog scores. The resulting groups were 15 male and 15 female dog lovers, and 15 male and 15 female dog-neutral subjects.

Comparison Studied

The purpose was to clarify which of three possible factors—cognition, conditioning, and tactual contact comfort—exerts the major influence in the so-called pet effect. Subjects with positive and neutral attitudes toward dogs had tactile, verbal, and verbal-tactile interaction with a dog while their HR and BP were recorded using a Dinamap. Subjects were given an opportunity to get acquainted with the dog and 20 minutes to adapt to the BP cuff cycle. Subjects were also exposed to two interview conditions, one with the dog present and one with the dog absent, and a rest condition with the dog absent from the room. The order of the exposure to the conditions was randomized and subjects were exposed to each of the conditions for a period of 6 minutes, with BP and HR recorded every 2 minutes.

Key Results

Blood pressure was significantly higher in the two interviews than in the verbal, verbal-tactile, tactile, and rest conditions. Blood pressure was also significantly lower in the tactile and rest conditions than in the verbal-tactile or verbal conditions. Heart rate was significantly higher in the verbal-tactile condition and significantly lower in the rest condition than in all other conditions.

Study Strengths and Weaknesses

This is a well-designed study with little threat to internal or external validity. Generalizability is limited to younger subjects free from known illness.

Clinical Implications

Results support the view that human interactions with a pet dog have a positive effect on BP. Touch appears to be the major component of the pet effect; cognitive factors contribute to a lesser degree.

6. Allen K, Shykoff BE, Isso JL, Jr. Pet ownership, but not ACE inhibitor therapy, blunts home blood pressure responses to mental stress. *Hypertension*. 2001;38(4):815-820.

Study Sample

Subjects were hypertensive patients (uncomplicated stage II+) with a high stress occupation (stockbroker). Of the 48 participants, 24 were men (18 white, 6 black) and 24 were women (18 white, 6 white). All were on home medication and seen in a physician's office.

Comparison Studied

The effect of pet ownership on blood pressure response to mental stress before and during ACE inhibitor therapy was evaluated.

Study Procedures

A pretest-posttest control group design was used. All subjects were interested in stress reduction and agreed to acquire a pet in randomized to the pet ownership group. Each group had 24 participants. Each participant had baseline mental stress sessions in their home after one month of observation. Stressors included mental arithmetic task and speech, both having been used in numerous studies to produce significant cardiovascular response. Heart rate, systolic blood pressure, and diastolic blood pressures were recorded once a minute throughout the experiment using a Propaq monitor. A questionnaire about social support was also completed. After baseline measures, later in the day, participants performed 2 psychologically stressful tasks in their home. HR, SBP and DBP were recorded once a minute during the tasks and Renin was assessed three times (after the initial rest, and after each stressful task). After this initial testing, they were treated

with lisinopril 20 mg/day. The pet ownership group acquired their pet at the time drug therapy began. A second mental stress evaluation occurred six months later in their home and again in the physician office. The experimental group performed the second evaluation in the presence of their pets.

Key Results

Before drug therapy, the mean responses to mental stress did not differ significantly between the two groups. Lisinopril therapy lowered resting blood pressure equally in both groups. However, blood pressure responses to mental stress were significantly lower ($P < .0001$) among pet owners. Conclusion: lisinopril only reduces blood pressure, and increased social support through pet ownership lowers blood pressure response to mental stress. Blood pressure readings in both groups were significantly higher in the office than in the home before and after both intervention therapy sessions.

Study Strengths and Weaknesses

This is a well designed study despite the small sample size. The sample was selected for its homogeneity, but this limits the generalization of the study findings as does the limitations due to the single setting. Because neither pet ownership nor lisinopril therapy controlled blood pressure measured in the physician office, it is logical to question the role of pet therapy in other stressful environments.

Clinical Implications

This study suggests that increased social support from pet ownership may enhance and complement medication therapy for hypertension. Assessing patients for the potential of this benefit can facilitate patient education.

OTHER REFERENCES

1. Brickel CM. A review of the roles of pet animals in psychotherapy and with the elderly. *Int J Aging Hum Dev*. 1980;12:119-128.
2. Grossberg JM, Alf EF Jr. Interaction with pet dogs: effects on human cardiovascular response. *J Delta Soc*. 1985;2(1):20-27.
3. Jorgensen, J. Therapeutic use of companion animals in health care. *Image J Nurs Schol*. 1997;29:249-254.
4. Martin, S. Ask the experts. *Crit Care Nurse*. 1993;13(2):74,79.
5. Messnet PR. Social facilitation of contact with other people by pet dogs. In: Katcher AH, Beck AM, eds. *New Perspectives on Our Lives With Companion Animals*. Philadelphia, Pa: University of Pennsylvania Press; 1983:37-46.
6. Plant M, Zimmerman EM, Goldstein RA. Health hazards to humans associated with domestic pets. *Annu Rev Public Health*. 1996;17:221-245.
7. Thoma LM. *Physiological Effects in the Hypertensive*

Individual of Petting Bonded vs Nonbonded Dogs [thesis]. Omaha, Neb: University of Nebraska Medical Center, College of Nursing; 1984.

8. Toss-Schulke ST, Trask B, Wallace C. *Petting a Companion Dog and Coronary Prone Behaviors: Effects on Systolic and Diastolic Blood Pressure, Heart Rate, and Peripheral Skin Temperature* [dissertation]. Omaha, Neb: University of Nebraska Medical Center, College of Nursing; 1988.

9. Wilson CC. Physiological responses of college students to a pet. *J Nerv Ment Dis.* 1987;175:606-612.

10. Wilson CC. The pet as an anxiolytic intervention. *J Nerv Ment Dis.* 1991;179:482-489.

11. Harvey MA, Ninos NP, Adler DC, et al. Results of the consensus conference on fostering more humane critical care: creating a healing environment. *AACN Clin Issues.* 1993;4(3):484-549.

12. Hooker SD, Freeman LH, Stewart P. Pet therapy research: a historical review. *Holist Nurs Pract.* 2002; 16(5):17-23.

13. Proulx D. Animal-assisted therapy. *Crit Care Nurs.* 1998; 18(2):81-84.

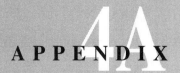

Sample Pet Visiting Forms

1. Consent for Participation in the Family Pet Visiting Program

Sample Form

HOSPITAL NAME
CITY, STATE

CONSENT FOR PARTICIPATION IN THE FAMILY PET VISIT PROGRAM

* *

I, _____, the patient/parent/legal guardian of _____

consent to my/his/her participation in _____ Hospital's Family Pet Visitation Program.

I understand that this program is designed to allow interaction between a patient and his/her pet. I

have been informed that I can bring the family pet to a specially designated area on the unit. I will

assure that the pet will be screened according to health standards and temperament.

   I have informed _____ Hospital that to my knowledge I/my dependent (circle one)

do not have/does not have allergies to this pet.

   My signature indicates that I have read this document and that I fully understand it.

_____   _____   _____
            Signature   Date & Time   Witness

_____

Source: Used with permission by the Family Intervention Research Team,
University of Iowa Hospitals and Clinics and the University of Iowa
College of Nursing, Iowa City, Iowa.

2. Family Pet Visiting Program Health Certificate

Sample Form

_____ **HOSPITAL**

FAMILY PET VISITATION PROGRAM HEALTH CERTIFICATE

All persons must turn in an up-to-date health certificate on the family pet *before* the pet will be allowed into the building. This form must be completed by a veterinarian not more than six months ago and must indicate that all immunizations are current and that the pet is free of ecto- and endoparasites. The health certificate is to be turned in to the nurse manager.

_____ Hospital requires this health certificate to protect the patient, other medical center guests, personnel, and the family pet.

* *

This is to certify that _____ owned by
(name of family pet)

_____ has been examined on _____ and was
(name of family member)   (date)

found to be free from disease, parasites, and is in good general health, temperament, is stable, and the animal is up to date on all recommended immunizations.

(Please list immunizations and dates below.)

Veterinarian's signature: _____

Address: _____

Telephone number: _____   Date: _____

_____

Source: Used with permission by the Family Intervention Research Team, University of Iowa Hospitals and Clinics and the University of Iowa College of Nursing, Iowa City, Iowa.

3. Release from Responsibility Waiver, Family Pet Visiting Program

Sample Form

_____ HOSPITAL

**RELEASE FROM RESPONSIBILITY WAIVER
FAMILY PET VISIT PROGRAM**

* *

I hereby absolve _____ Hospital and its personnel from any and all liability for any incidents which might injure a patient, visitor, or staff member as a result of my pet visiting _____ Hospital. I accept full responsibility for any damages my pet may incur and risks or injuries sustained by my pet while visiting at _____ Hospital. Attached is a health certificate signed by the pet's veterinarian certifying the pet's suitability for participation in this program.

I agree to abide by the policies and procedures set forth by the Family Pet Visitation program to ensure a _safe and pleasant visit by my pet._

Signed: _____   Date: _____

Telephone #: _____

Type of pet: _____

Pet owner's insurance carrier: _____

_____

Source: Used with permission by the Family Intervention Research Team, University of Iowa Hospitals and Clinics and the University of Iowa College of Nursing, Iowa City, Iowa.

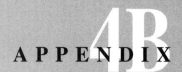
Resources for Animal-Assisted Activities and Animal-Assisted Therapy

1. Delta Society
   289 Perimeter Road East
   Renton, WA 98055-1329
   Phone: 1-800-869-6898
   E-mail: Deltasociety@CIS.Compuserve.Com
   Web site: http://www.deltasociety.com

2. Association for Practitioners in Infection Control (APIC)
   1016 16th Street NW, 6th Floor
   Washington, DC 20036
   Phone: (202) 296-2742

   This group is developing a standard infection control policy for pet therapy.

3. *Standards of Practice for Animal-assisted Activities and Therapy.* Renton, Wash: Delta Society; 1996.

4. Fredrickson, M. *Pet Partners Program. Introductory Handler Skills Course for Animal-assisted Activities and Therapy. Home Study Version.* 2nd ed. Renton, Wash: Delta Society; 1996.

Source: Used with permission by the Family Intervention Research Team, University of Iowa Hospitals and Clinics and the University of Iowa College of Nursing, Iowa City, Iowa.

Spiritual and Complementary Therapies to Promote Healing and Reduce Stress

Stephanie Woods, RN, PhD

Spiritual and Complementary Therapies to Promote Healing and Reduce Stress

CASE STUDIES: PATIENTS

Mr Jacobs, a 56-year-old certified public accountant who owns his own business, is admitted to the ICU. He has been experiencing episodes of a rapid and irregular pulse rate, palpitations, and dizziness. Because these episodes began during tax season, his busiest time, he did not seek medical care. Attributing his signs and symptoms to anxiety, he purchased an over-the-counter herbal preparation, kava, and has been taking the herbal daily to control his anxiety. He states this was helping his symptoms until last night. After a particularly stressful day, he became tachycardic and very dizzy, upon which his wife brought him to the emergency room. He was found to be in atrial fibrillation at rates between 120 to 160. His blood pressure was 84/60 upon admission. Admitted for rate control, stabilization of blood pressure, and anticoagulation, he asks if he can continue his kava for anxiety relief.

- Where would you access information regarding herbals such as kava? How would you determine the standard dose and dosing frequency?
- Where would you access information regarding drug-herbal and herbal-herbal interactions?

Mrs Harris is an 84-year-old female, admitted to the ICU for heart failure. She is well known to the staff due to numerous admissions in the past. Despite the acuity of the situation and her obvious discomfort, the nurse notes that Mrs Harris seems serenely calm. Once the patient's vital signs have stabilized and she becomes more comfortable, the nurse asks her how she can remain so peaceful during an acute exacerbation. Ms. Harris replies, "No matter the situation, I just pray. It is prayer that brings me through." The nurse also notes that when Mrs Harris prays with her pastor or family members, that her heart rate and blood pressure normalize.

- The patient asks the nurse to pray with her. Is it ethical for the nurse to do so?
- Is there evidence to support that prayer indeed can lower blood pressure and heart rate?

CASE STUDIES: STAFF

Samantha Allen has been a critical care nurse for 5 years. Her mother died recently with a myocardial infarction. Samantha blames herself for not recognizing signs and symptoms early and for not encouraging her mother to seek a thorough cardiac evaluation. Coworkers are concerned that Samantha is depressed. Samantha has also voiced concerns over inability to sleep, feelings of anxiety, and tearfulness since her mother's death. One of the staff nurses suggests that Samantha try herbal preparations such as Saint-John's-wort or melatonin to treat her symptoms. Another nurse suggests imagery and prayer as potential interventions. Samantha is unsure of the science behind these interventions and instead opts for traditional treatments of an antidepressant and psychotherapy.

- How can you determine the efficacy of herbal and botanicals?
- How do herbal and botanical products compare with traditional medications for the treatment of depression?

Joe Ramirez is a 30-year veteran on night shift in the surgical intensive care unit. He has smoked up to 2 packs of cigarettes per day since he was a young man. Recently he has begun taking antihypertensive medication and had some nonspecific changes on his EKG during a cardiac stress test. Motivated to improve his health, he decided to quit smoking.

He has undergone acupuncture treatments and has been able to stop smoking. Joe attributes his success to the acupuncture treatments and is recommending them to friends and colleagues who smoke.

- Is there any evidence to support success of acupuncture in smoking cessation?

This Protocol for Practice is designed to provide evidence-based information that can be easily integrated into patient care and staff interventions. Recommendations will be made based upon a review of the science related to complementary and alternative medicine. An extensive reference list will provide a basis for addressing patient and staff situations such as described in the case studies above.

GENERAL DESCRIPTION

Stress, Immunocompetence, and the Development of Disease

The term *stress* refers to a heightened physical or mental state produced in an organism by a change in the internal or external environment. The critical care environment is stressful for patients and staff (see Figure 5-1). In humans, physical stress is caused by injuries or illnesses, by psychological stress, or by perceived or anticipated threats.[1,2] When events such as hospitalization for a patient or environmental work conditions for a staff member are perceived as threatening by the higher cortical centers, signals are sent to the motor cortex and hypothalamus. Several hormones are released from the pituitary and adrenal glands, resulting in a number of physiological manifestations that can produce further harm to already compromised systems. For patients, the increased heart rate and work of breathing and increased oxygen consumption can have an adverse influence on patient outcome. For staff, job stress influences productivity, absenteeism, job turnover, satisfaction, and physical health. For both, the anxiety, fear, anger, or depression that often results from unmanaged stress is detrimental to the therapeutic relationship and to patients' outcomes. Figure 5-2 summarizes the stress response.[3] Any patient or staff member with subjective or objective signs of stress is a candidate for one or more stress-reduction therapies.

The relationship of stress to the decreased perception of wellness and subsequent development of disease is best described by an evolving field of study, psychoneuroimmunology. Psychoneuroimmunology studies the interactions between consciousness and perception (psychological), the brain and nervous system (neurological), and the body's defenses against infection and abnormal cell growth (immunology). Psychoneuroimmunology more fully relates the stress response to immunocompetence.

Stress and the impact on immunocompetence has been linked to the development of disease. Stress can lead to immunosuppression, thereby affecting development and progression of disease. Evidence supports that the degree of stress is related to the rates of respiratory tract infections, malignancy, and resistance to metastasis.[1,2,4,5] Additionally, stress and immunocompetence have been studied in patients with AIDs, cardiovascular disease, and depression. Although only a few prospective, randomized, controlled clinical trials have been conducted in this new area of study, such studies are increasing.

The psychoneuroimmunology system is activated by cues. These cues can be visual (seeing a snake), cognitive (knowing that snakes often inhabit woodland paths such as the one you are walking along), physical (feeling something cold alongside your foot), and emotional (feeling fearful when you see a snake while walking along a woodland path). No matter how the system is cued, a cascade of physiological events occurs (see Figure 5-2). Although the stress response is designed to be protective, Figure 5-2 demonstrates that the negative impact of stress on the immune system can result in decreased immune response and ultimately development of disease and abnormal cellular replication.

Many forms of complimentary and alternative medicine are used to reduce stress and anxiety, thereby reducing negative stimulation of the psychoneuroimmunology system. The anticipated result is ultimately prevention of or reduction in illness, symptom mediation, and improved state of well-being.

Definitions

Complimentary and alternative medicine (CAM) is defined as "a group of diverse medical and health care systems, practices, and products that are not presently considered to be part of conventional medicine, that is, medicine as practiced by holders of medical doctor or doctor of osteopathy degrees and their allied health professionals such as physical therapists, psychologists, and registered nurses."[6] What constitutes alternative or complementary care depends on the current standard of medical practice. For example, hypnosis and dietary therapies were once considered outside the mainstream but are now part of accepted medical practice. As scientific evidence demonstrates the efficacy of CAM, these practices are incorporated into conventional health care.

Acknowledgement of the practice of CAM by consumers, and the acceptance of CAM as a treatment option, was evident by the establishment of the Office of Alternative Medicine (OAM), a part of the National Institutes of Health (NIH) in 1991. The goals of the office were to (1) facilitate the evaluation of alternative treatment modalities, (2) investigate and evaluate the efficacy of alternative treatments, (3) establish an information clearinghouse to exchange information with the public about alternative medicine, and (4) support research training in alternative practices.

In 1999, the OAM became an independent component of NIH and was renamed the National Center for Complementary and Alternative Medicine (NCCAM). The NCCAM Information Clearinghouse was established in 1996. In 1997, the first phase 3 clinical trials for CAM were done to study

Figure 5-1   Stresses in the acute and critical care environment

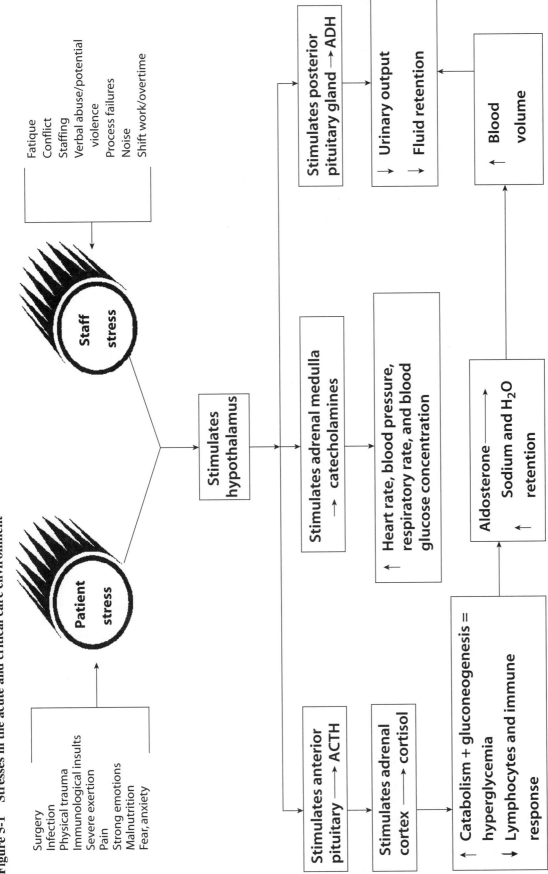

Surgery
Infection
Physical trauma
Immunological insults
Severe exertion
Pain
Strong emotions
Malnutrition
Fear, anxiety

Fatigue
Conflict
Staffing
Verbal abuse/potential violence
Process failures
Noise
Shift work/overtime

Patient stress

Staff stress

Stimulates hypothalamus

Stimulates anterior pituitary $\longrightarrow$ ACTH

Stimulates adrenal cortex $\longrightarrow$ cortisol

Catabolism + gluconeogenesis = hyperglycemia
$\uparrow$ Lymphocytes and immune response

Stimulates adrenal medulla $\longrightarrow$ catecholamines

$\uparrow$ Heart rate, blood pressure, respiratory rate, and blood glucose concentration

Stimulates posterior pituitary gland $\longrightarrow$ ADH

$\uparrow$ Urinary output
$\uparrow$ Fluid retention

Aldosterone $\longrightarrow$ Sodium and H_2O retention

$\uparrow$ Blood volume

Figure 5-2 The stress response. *Notes:* ACTH, adrenocorticotropic hormone; ADH, antidiuretic hormone; PMNs, polymorphonuclear leukocytes; RNA, ribonucleic acid.

From: Shelby J, McCance K. Stress and disease. In: McCance K, Huether S, eds. *Pathophysiology: The Biologic Basis for Disease in Adults and Children.* Fourth ed. St. Louis: Mosby; 2002:283-284.

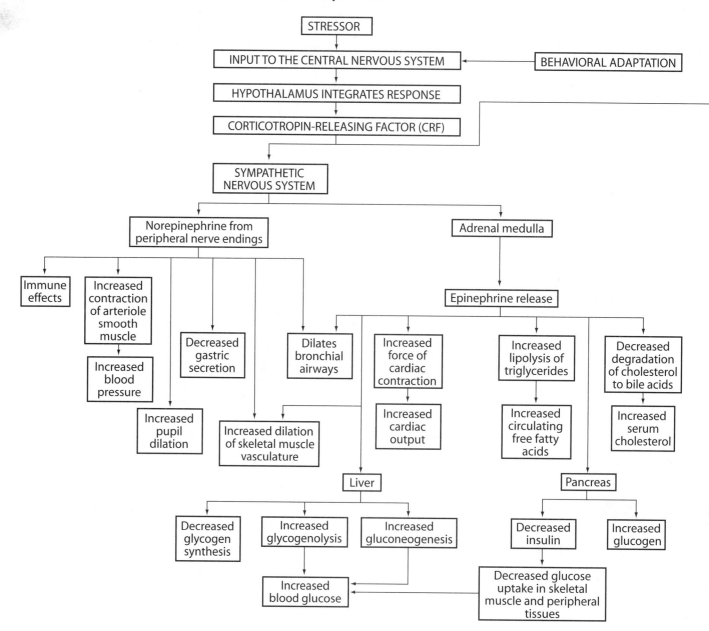

the efficacy of Saint-John's-wort in clinical depression.[7] In 1999, the first NCAAM research awards were granted. Ten clinical research centers with the mission to conduct research related to alternative therapies have been established around the country. At this time, NCCAM is supporting approximately 300 ongoing research projects.

The NCCAM is dedicated to improving the science of complementary and alternative medicine and consequently the health of those consumers who use CAM. The 2005-2009 NCCAM Strategic Plan[6] sets goals that will further science in the CAM domains and practices that have the greatest ability to do the following:

- Enhance physical and mental health and wellness.
- Manage pain and other symptoms, disabilities, and functional impairment.

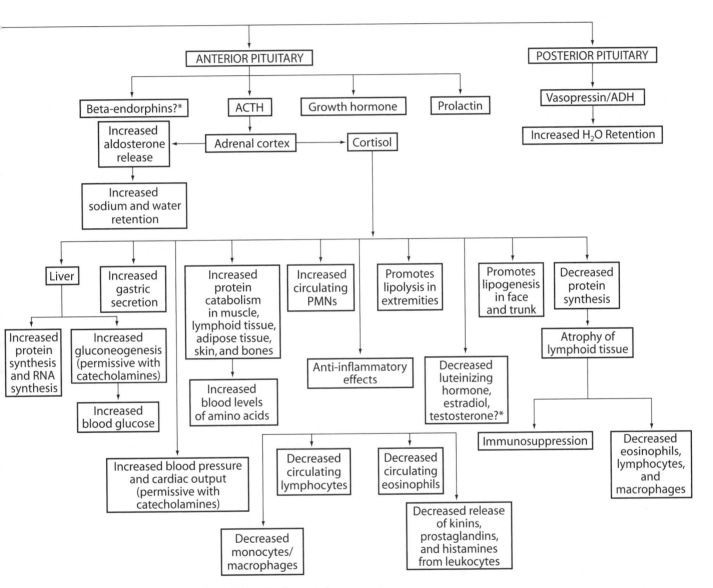

*Unclear whether endorphins originate from pituitary gland or central nervous system.

- Significantly affect a specific disease or disorder.
- Prevent disease and empower the public to take responsibility for their health.
- Reduce selected health problems of specific populations.

Complementary medicine is used *in conjunction with* conventional medicine. Alternative medicine is used *instead of* conventional medicine. Common CAM practices are part of whole medical systems. Whole medical systems are based on beliefs and principles that are very different, even contrary, to traditional medicine. Whole medical systems are most often associated with ancient medical systems such as traditional Chinese medicine (TCM) and Ayurvedic medicine from India. Homeopathy and naturopathy are also included in whole medical systems. The commonality of these systems is that they are individualized to the patient's needs and use multiple modes of therapy. For instance, whole systems use general modalities found in many of the four CAM domains, such as diet, exercise, and lifestyle modification in addition to specific modalities found within the domains, such as acupuncture.

NCCAM identifies the following 4 domains of CAM practices:

- Mind-body medicine, which includes yoga, meditation, the placebo effect, and prayer
- Biologically based practices using herbal, botanical, and other natural products. These products can include vitamins, minerals, and probiotics. Diets considered healthful are also included in these practices.
- Manipulative and body-based practices, including chiropractic and osteopathic manipulation and massage
- Energy medicine involves the use of verifiable sources of energy that are thought to impart healing energies. These energies include electromagnetic radiation, sound, and biofields.

The National Center for Complimentary and Alternative Medicine and the National Center for Health Statistics, part of the Centers for Disease Control and Prevention (CDC), recently published the most recent National Health Interview Survey. This survey details American's health and illness-related experiences. Data was collected in 2002 from 31,044 adults aged 18 or older. The survey queried participants regarding their use of commonly used CAM therapies. Thirty-six percent of US adults use some form of CAM. When megavitamin use and prayer are included in the definition of CAM, this percentage rises to 62%. The survey found that most surveyed used CAM *along with* conventional medicine versus *instead of* conventional medicine. CAM was most frequently used to prevent or treat musculoskeletal conditions associated with chronic or recurring pain.

Considerations Related to the Use of Alternative Therapies

The use of CAM practices is largely unregulated and usually not prescribed by health care practitioners. Despite this, consumers are using complementary and alternative therapies in increasing numbers. The most recent data available from 1997 showed that Americans spent an estimated $36-47 billion on CAM therapies. Of that amount, between $12 and $20 billion was paid for services of CAM practitioners or professionals. These service fees represent more than the public paid out of pocket for all hospitalizations in 1997, and approximately 50% for all out-of-pocket expenses for conventional MD/DO visits.[8,9]

A recent survey of 776 critical care nurses, all members of the American Association of Critical-Care Nurses, demonstrated that complementary or alternative therapies are commonly used in the practice of critical-care nurses. The survey listed 28 select practices, organized according to the 4 domains of mind-body practices, biologicals, manipulative body-

based practices, and energy medicine. A consistent pattern of use in professional practice was found across the 5 geographical regions of the United States. Similar patterns were found as well for personal use of practices across geographical regions. A majority of nurses were open to learning more and increasing use of alternative practices in their care of patients. Practices such as massage, exercise, diet, relaxation, prayer, and counseling were found to be most commonly used. Native American and traditional Chinese medicine were among the least used practices.[10]

A growing body of evidence indicates that alternative therapies, either by themselves or in combination with conventional medical treatment, are effective. For example, in one study, meditation combined with guided imagery decreased body tension, emotional anxiety, and the adverse physical effects of chemotherapy.[11] At the University of California, Dean Ornish showed that coronary heart disease actually can be reversed with nutrition, exercise, and meditation without the use of medication or surgery.[12,12-14]

Complementary or alternative therapies may be used and integrated into the general treatment plan more effectively when the conventional practitioner is aware of the client's use of these practices. Many patients do not confide their use of alternative therapies to their mainstream medical practitioner. Some therapies may support and enhance conventional treatments, but others have the potential for untoward effects. To prevent harm to patients, conventional practitioners should carefully assess the use of alternative therapies by their clients.

Complementary Therapies for Reducing Stress and Anxiety

It is not the purpose of this protocol to debate the East versus West approach to healing, nor the safety or efficacy of traditional medicine versus CAM practices. Practitioners and consumers of CAM cite centuries of evidence for safety and efficacy of their practices. Indeed, consumers' buying patterns and accessing of CAM practices suggest a strong propensity to integrate the domains and specific practices of CAM with or without evidence for safety or efficacy. It is the individual right of consumers to pursue their choice in integration of CAM practices into their personal health care choices.

Health care professionals may find searching for scientific evidence for CAM practices frustrating. The special language of CAM and varying indexing techniques in the databases can make it difficult to adequately search and find evidence to support use of the various practices. Although resources for CAM information are increasing, it can be challenging to identify authoritative sources. Health care professionals may have trouble isolating the existent knowledge necessary to guide practice. When practitioners utilize the mainstream sources for health care information, such as MEDLINE, searches may end up being limited and superficial.[15]

Available systematic reviews and meta-analyses in the CAM literature were used in the preparation of this research protocol. Systematic reviews of the literature provide a reliable tool for summarizing evidence and efficacy of mainstream treatments.[16,17] However, for the practitioner interested in CAM practices, the utilization of systematic reviews may prove challenging. The steps authors follow in planning, performing, and interpreting literature in a systematic review may lead to divergent results. Although the intent of the systematic review is to reduce bias and make conclusions objective, the quality of the review is greatly dependent upon the quality of the primary sources and the quality of the review.[18] "Unless the results are very clear cut, reviewers with different prejudices about the hypothesis under investigation may draw different conclusions from the same data."[19] Indeed prejudice of Western reviewers of CAM practices has long been alleged, leading to disparaging reviews of CAM research.

There is evidence to support that the best conducted clinical trials provide the least promising results. This is because of reductionist methods and the focus on controlling variance thereby limiting definitive conclusions regarding effect. Limitations in systematically reviewing CAM literature include lack of a controlled vocabulary for CAM practices, underrepresentation of CAM literature in the mainline databases, mixtures of quantitative and qualitative approaches, and differences in inclusion criteria. Additionally, limiting searches to English-only literature excludes much of the relevant CAM literature.

Despite these limitations, the professional nurse must be responsible to consumers in his or her care. In support of professional practice, and to limit liability, this protocol focuses on CAM practices for which evidence supports safety and efficacy. Additionally, practices such as therapeutic touch and acupuncture that should be practiced by certified practitioners are not included.

Although many CAM therapies are being used in health care today, this protocol is limited to those specifically used to reduce stress and anxiety.

Most of the therapies discussed here can be independently instituted, but should be disclosed to the team of health care providers caring for the patient.

Commonly used care interventions, grouped under the 4 domains identified by NCCAM, have been chosen from hundreds of potential CAM practices. These practices have been selected based upon prevalence of use, practical application in the critical and acute care environment, and research data available.

Mind-Body Medicine

Mind-body medicine is the most frequently practiced form of CAM and involves the interaction of mind, brain, and body systems. Practices within this domain include tai chi, yoga, meditation, imagery, spiritual practices, and prayer. Mind-body medicine has been used to help patients with chronic diseases and terminal illnesses to improve the quality of life, achieve symptom relief, and improve outcomes. Yoga and meditation have been shown to be helpful in lowering of blood pressure and heart rate.[20] Meditation has also been associated with improved antibody response to flu vaccine.[21] Optimism and positive attitude have been related to increased longevity and more rapid recovery after cardiac transplant, further validating the interactions between mind and body.[22] Prayer has been linked to positive effects on recovery from alcoholism, depression, coping with stress, and quality of life.[23]

Mind-body practices focused on in this protocol are imagery and prayer.

Imagery

Imagery is a nonverbal, noninvasive intervention that can be implemented by patients alone or with guidance. Imagery uses the internal experiences of memories, dreams, fantasies, and visions to serve as the bridge for connecting body, mind, and spirit. As nurses gain an understanding of the effectiveness of imagery, they can use it to complement traditional nursing interventions. Guided imagery plus relaxation is being used with increased frequency to help persons improve their performance and control their responses to stressful situations. Relaxation and imagery are often used together because the use of images can assist in achieving relaxation, and relaxation helps foster the visualization of images.

Prayer

The relationship of religion, religious activity, and spirituality to health and healing has been widely researched and remains highly controversial. Despite methodological flaws, the growing body of evidence demonstrates a positive relationship between religious activities, such as attending church and prayer, with reduced mortality.[24-26] Other studies have shown a correlation between religious beliefs and practice and the sense of well-being.[27,28] Harold Koenig, psychiatrist and religious researcher, describes religion as a benefit package that includes health behaviors, lifestyle decisions, social and psychological connections, and a belief system that pulls the benefits together. However, others maintain that equal benefits can be obtained from counseling, joining social groups, and practicing healthful habits.[24]

Prayer is usually considered a religious or spiritual act. Prayer is generally defined as asking for something for oneself or others, from a higher power, often conceptualized as God. Intercessory prayer, the study of which frequently appears in the literature is defined as "organized, regular and committed, and those who practice it will almost inevitably hold some committed belief that they are praying to God."[29] Evidence exists that prayer has a positive effect on humans, mice, chicks, enzymes, bacteria, fungi, and tissues of various sorts.[30] Still many researchers posit that prayer simply elicits the placebo response. But, if prayer's efficacy were due to the placebo effect, would that necessarily invalidate the effects?

Many clinicians and researchers question if prayer should be studied at all.[31] Citing experts in research validity, the construct validity of prayer is challenged[32] as well as the adequacy of the construct for scientific investigation.[33] Some even assert that it is not religion or prayer that is being put to the test, but rather God.[31,34,35,36]

Detractors believe it is premature, perhaps even unethical, to advocate the practice of religion and/or prayer. These dissenting opinions persist despite numerous studies among priests, nuns, Jews, and people professing to be religious that demonstrate lesser mortality rates and greater health benefits.[37-39] Criticisms include lack of control for confounding variables, researcher bias and lack of construct validity, weak to nonexistent theoretical underpinnings, and methodological inadequacies[40] Dossey in his thoughtful review of prayer, *Healing Words,* states that not only can prayer be studied, it should be studied.[41] He states that while prayer does not need science to legitimize it, science can add to the understanding of the phenomenon.

Biologically Based Practices

Biologically based practices come from the natural world. Sources of healing have been identified in plant and animal extracts. Herbs, botanicals, select bacteria, and various diets touting their health benefit are popular among consumers. Herbal products marketed as dietary supplements are among the most popular CAM therapies in the United States. Clinical trials to test efficacy have proven difficult due to lack of quality controls within the dietary supplement industry. Many herbals fail to meet standards regarding purity and dosage.[42] Diets also create complex challenges to study as individual and cultural preferences often vary in approach.

Biologically based practices focused on in this protocol are herbals known to be effective in the relief of stress and anxiety, depression, and sleeplessness. Although these herbals must be prescribed by a physician if used in the hospitalized patient, they may be taken at will by staff. Caution must be taken to avoid drug interactions.

Of the 10 most commonly used biological preparations, only 4 have been found to have statistically significant evidence of efficacy in systematic reviews. These 4 biologicals are garlic, *Ginkgo biloba,* saw palmetto, and Saint-John's-wort.[42] Additionally, the hormone melatonin has been found to aid in sleep disorders secondary to jet lag.[43] Kava extract also appears to be effective in treating the symptoms of anxiety. However, safety issues have been cited in long-term kava[44] and melatonin use.[45] The biologically based compounds focused on in this protocol are melatonin, kava, and Saint-John's-wort.

Melatonin is a natural hormone produced by the pineal gland in the brain. Melatonin in part regulates the sleep cycle. The hormone levels rise markedly in the evening, causing drowsiness and facilitating sleep. In the morning, hormone levels fall, increasing wakefulness. Melatonin has been used by consumers to combat jet lag and to induce daytime sleep for night-shift workers. In a press release from the US Agency for Healthcare Research and Quality dated December 8, 2004, scientific evidence regarding melatonin effectiveness was reviewed.[43] In this review, melatonin supplements were found to have little benefit in jet lag and in inducing sleep for night-shift workers. The authors found evidence to suggest that short-term use of melatonin is safe and may help in resynchronizing the internal biological clock in delayed sleep phase syndrome. Delayed sleep phase syndrome makes it difficult to fall asleep until late at night and to awaken early. Melatonin supplements may also decrease sleep latency, the time it takes to fall asleep, in persons with insomnia. Melatonin does not seem to impact sleep efficiency, or the percentage of time a person is asleep after going to bed, in people with primary sleep disorders such as insomnia. Melatonin does not seem to impact sleep latency in people with secondary sleep disorders (from such disorders as mental illness, psychoses, mood and anxiety disorders, dementia, and Parkinson's), but does increase sleep efficiency modestly.

In a systematic review on melatonin and the prevention and treatment of jet lag, authors Herxheimer and Petrie came to different conclusions regarding the usefulness of melatonin for jet lag.[43] They found that melatonin was safe and very effective in preventing or reducing the effects of jet lag. They went on to recommend that melatonin be recommended to adult travelers who are prone to jet lag and who are flying across five or more time zones, particularly in an easterly direction. A potential interaction of melatonin with warfarin was cited, as was a contraindication of melatonin use in people with epilepsy. Additional research was recommended for these patient populations.[45]

The research on melatonin is incomplete and conflicting, therefore restricting firm conclusions regarding the usefulness of melatonin for sleep disorders. Continued research is necessary to prove or disprove efficacy and safety.

Biologically based practices are widely used for the reduction and treatment of anxiety. Kava, a biological created from the oceanic plant *Piper methysticum Forst,* is used by consumers to prevent and treat anxiety. In the year 2000, kava was among the top-selling herbs in the United States.[46] Several nonrandomized, noncontrolled studies have suggested that kava is beneficial in the treatment of anxiety.[47] Pittler and Ernst[48] found kava versus placebo use resulted in a significant reduction in anxiety as reported in the total score on the Hamilton-Anxiety (HAM-A) instrument. In a systematic review of kava extract for treating anxiety, meta-analysis of 6 trials suggested a significant treatment effect of kava on the total score on the Hamilton-Anxiety instrument. Few adverse events were reported in the use of kava, and all were mild, transient, and infrequent. The data from the systematic review found kava to be superior to placebo for the symptomatic treatment of anxiety.

On March 25, 2002, the U.S. Food and Drug Administration (FDA) issued a Consumer Advisory in which it advised "consumers of the potential risk of severe liver injury associated with the use of kava-containing dietary supplements." At the time of this consumer advisory, 68 cases of suspected kava hepatotoxicity were on record worldwide. Hepatic symptoms usually occurred 2-3 months after kava use. Most patients recovered fully, however 6 patients required liver transplantation and 3 died. Consumers who have known liver disease, drink alcohol, or have hepatic symptoms should not use kava.[44]

Saint-John's-wort, also known as *Hypericum perforatum,* is a biological used to elevate mood. The Hypericum Depression Trial Study Group was the first randomized controlled trial (RCT) conducted by the NCCAM.[7] Results published in 2003 found that Saint-John's-wort was no more effective than placebo or sertraline for treatment of major depression of moderate severity. There is an ongoing study to determine the value of Saint-John's-wort in treatment of minor depression.

Researchers outside of the NCCAM challenge the conclusions of the NCCAM-sponsored Hypericum Depression Trial Study.[49,50] Kirsch et al analyzed the clinical trial data submitted to the FDA to gain approval of 6 widely prescribed antidepressants. All data included the same depression measure, the Hamilton depression scale. Data was pooled across the various trials, and clinical as well as statistical significance was analyzed. In the analysis of this data, an 82% drug response to antidepressants was replicated in the placebo control groups. Simply put, participants receiving antidepressant medications and those who received placebos both improved significantly on total scores on the Hamilton depression scale.[51] So does placebo effect equal drug or biologicals effect in depression? More research is necessary to answer this important question.

Manipulative and Body-Based Practices

Manipulative and body-based practices are primarily accessed via the services of chiropractors, osteopaths, and massage therapists. These hands-on techniques are used to treat musculoskeletal conditions, asthma, and chronic pain. In the chiropractic literature, spinal manipulation is linked to alteration of nearby nerve cell tissue that is hypothesized to change circulating neurochemical and protein levels and nervous system function. Massagelike stimulation in animals has shown a release of morphine-like chemicals and relief of pain.[52] Chiropracty, osteopathic manipulation, massage, reflexology, and craniosacral therapy are body-based practices.

The manipulative and body-based practice focused on in this protocol is massage.

Massage
Massage is one of the numerous touch interventions designed to reduce stress, alleviate anxiety, promote circulation, and generally stimulate a feeling of well-being. Healing through the medium of touch is as old as civilization itself. The fact that all cultures have developed some form of touch therapy indicates that rubbing, pressing, massaging, and holding are natural manifestations of humans' desire to heal and care for one another. In the intervention of massage, the practitioner uses the 4 primary back care massage strokes to touch, push, knead, or rub the patient's skin and underlying tissue. The basic massage strokes of effleurage (with 2 stroking positions), pétrissage, and tapotement are listed and described in Appendix 5A.

Energy Medicine

Energy medicine is based on a belief that all living things have, transmit, and are affected by other's energy. This life energy, when decreased or imbalanced, is believed to lead to disease. This is verifiable by diagnostic tests such as electrocardiograms and electroencephalograms. External energies also appear to be helpful, such as electromagnetic fields and light energy. The study of energy medicine is impeded by the lack of measures and technology in the physical sciences. For example, current measures and technology are unavailable for validation of energy emitted by "healers" or practitioners of therapeutic touch.

No energy medicine practices are included in this protocol due to lack of instruments to confirm or deny safety and efficacy.

REVIEW OF SCIENTIFIC EVIDENCE FOR DOMAINS AND SELECT PRACTICES

Tables 5-1 through 5-5 provide a quick overview of the CAM domains, practices within the domain, goals for research within the domain, and potential metrics and levels of research required to expand current knowledge related to that domain.

Following the tables is an overview of current evidence organized by domain and select practices. Finally, a reference list is appended that is inclusive of classic and current literature for CAM in general and for each domain.

COMPETENCY

Nurses who offer complementary therapies should be trained in the use of the therapies. Numerous universities and agencies offer continuing education courses on selected CAM practices. Some schools of nursing incorporate some of the therapies in their skills courses.

Table 5-1 Research Needs in the Area of Whole Medical Systems

Whole Medical Systems	Goals for Research	Metrics	Levels of Research Needed
Traditional Chinese medicine Ayurvedic Homeopathy Naturopathy	Acquire a richer understanding of whole medicine systems. Conduct efficacy studies. Explore mechanisms of action in multimodal treatments in whole medical systems. Conduct multidisciplinary research.	Subjective Patient specific measures	Preclinical (bench) levels I-III, RCTs

Table 5-2 Research Needs in the Area of Mind-Body Practices

Mind-Body Practices	Goals for Research	Metrics	Levels of Research Needed
Tai chi Yoga Meditation Prayer	Explore the mechanisms of action for these practices. Explore the effects of these practices on stress reduction. Determine if these practices enhance resilience and ability to cope with illness and increase sense of wellness. Study the relationship of spirituality to health and healing.	Subjective Biochemical markers Brain imaging Immune assays and microflora Patient-specific measures	In vitro, tissue, and animal studies, preclinical (bench) levels I-III, RCTs

Table 5-3 Research Needs in the Area of Biologically Based Practices

Biologically Based Practices	Goals for Research	Metrics	Levels of Research Needed
Herbs and botanicals Pre- and probiotics Diets Bioactive compounds	Explore the mechanisms of biological action. Determine safety: • Purity and uniformity • Dosage • Efficacy • Verify, define composition • Therapeutic dose Determine pharmaceutical and pharmocokinetic properties. Explore efficacy in maintaining health, preventing disease, and treating conditions.	Biochemical markers DNA microassay proteomics Immune assays and microflora Drug interactions between drug-herbals, herbal-herbal	In vitro, tissue, and animal studies, preclinical (bench) levels I-III, RCTs

Table 5-4 Research Needs in the Area of Manipulative and Body-Based Practices

Manipulative and Body-Based Practices	Goals for Research	Metrics	Levels of Research Needed
Chiropracty Osteopathic Manipulation Massage Reflexology Craniosacral therapy	Explore the mechanisms of action for these practices. Determine disorders and states of wellness that are benefited by these practices. Formulate optimal regimens. Determine the cost-benefit of such practices.	Subjective reports of outcomes (wellness, improved function) Biochemical markers for pain, patient ratings of pain MRI, PET scan data Measures of tissue strain and neurological, immunological, and endocrine responses	In vitro, tissue, and animal studies, preclinical (bench) levels I-III

Table 5-5 Research Needs in the Area of Energy Medicine Practices

Energy Medicine Practices	Goals for Research	Metrics	Levels of Research Needed
Qi gong Therapeutic touch Reiki Polarity Healing touch Johrei	Apply the rigor of accepted clinical research to energy medicine. Conduct multidisciplinary research, pairing basic scientists, CAM, and non-CAM practitioners	Few measurement devices exist to confirm the energy said to be transmitted by the various energy medicine practices.	Preclinical models, standardization of methods, placebo effects, study characteristics of practitioners

REFERENCE LIST

1. Selye H. *The Stress of Life.* New York, NY: McGraw-Hill; 1956.
2. Cannon WB. *The Wisdom of the Body.* New York, NY: Norton; 1932.
3. Shelby J, McCance K. Stress and disease. In: McCance K, Huether S, eds. *Pathophysiology: The Biologic Basis for Disease in Adults and Children.* 4th ed. St. Louis, Mo: Mosby; 2002.
4. Lengacher C, Bennet M, Gonzalez L, Cox C. Psychoneuroimmunology and immune system link for stress, depression health behaviors, and breast cancer. *Altern Health Pract.* 1999;2:95-108.
5. Caine R. Psychological influences in critical care: perspectives from psychoneuroimmunology. *Crit Care Nurse.* 2003;23:60-69.
6. National Center for Complementary and Alternative Medicine (NCCAM). *Strategic Plan 2005-2009.* Washington, DC: NCCAM; 2004.
7. Hypericum Depression Trial Study Group. Effect of Hypericum perforattum (St. John's wort) in major depressive disorder: a randomized controlled trial. *JAMA.* 2003;290:1500-1504.
8. Barnes P, Powell-Griner E, McFann K, Nahin R. *CDC Advance Data Report #343.* Complementary and alternative medicine use among adults: United States, 2002. May 27, 2004. Available at: http://nccam.nih.gov/news/camstats.htm. Accessed November 8, 2006.
9. Eisenberg D, Davis R, Ettner S, et al. Trends in alternative medicine use in the United States, 1990-1997. *JAMA.* 1998;280:1569-1575.
10. Lindquist R, Tracy M, Savik K, Watanuki S. Regional use of complementary and alternative therapies by critical care nurses. *Crit Care Nurse.* 2005;25:63-75.
11. Thomson B. Alternative therapies. *Nat Health.* 1992; 68-69.
12. Ornish D. Can lifestyle changes reverse coronary heart disease? *Lancet.* 1990;336:129.
13. Ornish D. Lessons from the Lifestyle Heart Trial. *Choices Cardiol.* 1991;1:1-4.
14. Ornish D. Can lifestyle changes reverse coronary heart disease? *World Rev Nutr Diet.* 1993;72:38-48.
15. Owen D, Fang M. Information-seeking behavior in complementary and alternative medicine: an online survey of faculty at a health sciences campus. *J Med Libr Assoc.* 2003;91:311-321.
16. Chalmers I, Altman D, eds. *Systematic Reviews.* London: BMJ Publishing Group; 1995.
17. Cook D, Mulrow C, Haynes R. Systematic reviews: synthesis of best evidence for clinical decisions. *Ann Intern Med.* 1997;126:376-380.
18. Schulz K, Chalmers I, Hayes R, Altman D. Empirical evidence of bias. *JAMA.* 1995;274:1942-1948.
19. Linde K, Willich S. How objective are systematic reviews? Differences between reviews on complementary medicine. *JR Soc Med.* 2003;96:17-22.
20. Schmidt T, Wijga A, Von Zur Muhle A, et al. Changes in cardiovascular risk factors and hormones during a comprehensive residential three month Kriya yoga training and vegetarian nutrition. *Acta Physiol Scand Suppl.* 1997;640:158-162.
21. Davidson R, Kabat-Zinn J, Schumacher J, et al. Alterations in brain and immune function produced by mindfulness meditation. *Psychosom Med.* 2003;65:564-570.
22. Danner D, Snowdon D, Friesen W. Positive emotions in early life and longevity: findings from the nun study. *J Pers Soc Psychol.* 2001;80:804-813.
23. Matthews D, McCullough M, Larson D, Koenig H, Swyers J, Milano M. Religious commitment and health status. *Arch Family Medicine.* 1998;7:118-24.
24. Koenig H, Hays JC, Larson D, et al. Does religious attendance prolong survival? A six year follow-up study of 3,968 older adults. *J Gerontol Med Sci.* 1999;54A: M370-M377.
25. Orman D, Reed D. Religion and mortality among the community-dwelling elderly. *Am J Public Health.* 1998; 88:1469-1475.
26. House J, Robbins C, Metsner H. The association of social relationships and activities with mortality: prospective evidence from the Tecumseh Community Health Study. *Am J Epidemiol.* 1982;116:123-140.
27. Koenig H, Kvale J, Ferrel C. Religion and well-being in later life. *Gerontologist.* 1998;28:18-28.
28. Ellison C. Religious involvement and subjective well-being. *J Health Social Behav.* 1991;32:80-99.

29. Roberts L, Ahmed I, Hall S. Intercessory prayer for the alleviation of ill health [online]. *The Cochrane Database of Systematic Reviews: Reviews 2000.* Amended October, 2003; Article No. CD000368. Available at: http://www.update-software.com/Abstracts/AB000368.htm. Accessed November 8, 2006.

30. Benor D. Survey of spiritual healing research. *Complement Med Res.* 1990;4:9-33.

31. Chibnall J, Jeral J, Cerullo M. Experiments on distant intercessory prayer: God, science, and the lesson massah. *Arch Intern Med.* 2001;161:2529-2536.

32. Cook T, Campbell D. *Quasi-Experimentation: Design and Analysis Issues for Field Settings.* Boston, Mass: Houghton Mifflin Co; 1979.

33. Hempel CG. *Philosophy of Natural Science.* Englewood Cliffs, NJ: Prentice-Hall International Inc; 1990.

34. Sloan R, Bagiella E. Data without a prayer [letter]. *Arch Intern Med.* 2000;26:1870.

35. Galishoff M. God, prayer, and coronary care unit outcomers: faith vs. works [letter]. *Arch Intern Med.* 2000; 26:1877.

36. Hammerschmidt D. Ethical and practical problems in studying prayer [letter]. *Arch Intern Med.* 2000;26: 1874-1875.

37. Michalek A, Mettlin C, Priore R. Prostate cancer mortality among Catholic priests. *Surg Oncol.* 1981;17:129-133.

38. Timio M, Lippi G, Venanzi S, et al. Blood pressure trend and cardiovascular events in nuns in a secluded order: a 30-year follow-up study. *Blood Press.* 1997;6:81-87.

39. Goldbourt U, Yaari S, Medalie JH. Factors predictive of long-term coronary heart disease mortality among 10,059 male Israeli civil servants and municipal employees. *Cardiology.* 1993;82:100-121.

40. Sloan R, Bagiella E, Powell T. Religion, spirituality, and medicine. *Lancet.* 1999;353:664-667.

41. Dossey L. *Healing Words: The Power of Prayer and the Practice of Medicine.* New York, NY: Harper San Francisco; 1995.

42. Bent S, Ko R. Commonly used herbal medicines in the United States: a review. *Am J Med.* 2004;116:478-485.

43. Herxheimer A, Petrie K. Melatonin for the prevention and treatment of jet lag. *BMJ* 2003;326:296-297.

44. Consumer Advisory Center for Food Safety and Applied Nutrition, US Food and Drug Administration. Kava-containing dietary supplements may be associated with severe liver injury. Available at: http://www.cfsan.fda.gov/%7Edms/addskava.html. Accessed November 8, 2006.

45. Agency for Healthcare Research and Quality. *AHRQ Issues New Report on the Safety and Effectiveness of Melatonin Supplements.* Rockville, Md: AHRQ; 2004.

46. Blumenthal, M. Herb sales down 15 percent in mainstream market. *Herbalgram* 2001;51:69.

47. Pittler M, Ernst E. Kava extract for treating anxiety. Cochrane Database Syst Rev. 2003;(1):CD003383. Available at: http://www.update-software.com/abstracts/ab003383.htm. Accessed November 8, 2006.

48. Pittler M, Ernst E. Efficacy of kava extract for treating anxiety: systematic review and meta-analysis. *J Clin Psychoparmacol.* 2000;20:84-89.

49. Kirsch, I. St. John's Wort, conventional medication, and placebo: an egregious double standard. *Comp Ther Med.* 2003;11:193-195.

50. Linde L, Ramirez G, Multow CD, Weidenhammer W, Melchart D. St. John's wort for depression: an overview and meta-analysis of randomized clinical trials. *Br Med J.* 1996;313:253-258.

51. Kirsch I, Moore TJ, Scoboria A, Nicholls SS. The emperor's new drugs: an analysis of antidepressant medication data submitted to the FDA. Available at: http://www.journals.apa.org/prevention/volume5/pre0050023a.html. Accessed November 8, 2006.

52. Lund I, Yu L, Uvnas-Moberg K, et al. Repeated massage-like stimulation induces long-term effect of nociception; contribution of oxytocinergic mechanisms. *Eur J Neurosci.* 2002;16:330-338.

SUGGESTED READING

1. Snyder M. An overview of complementary/alternative therapies. In: Snyder M, Lindquist R, eds. *Complementary/Alternative Therapies in Nursing.* 4th ed. New York, NY: Springer; 2002:3-15.

2. Lu K. Herb use in critical care: what to watch for. *Crit Care Nurs Clin North Am.* 2003;15:313-319.

3. Sparber A. Complementary therapy in critical care settings: a review of surveys and implications for nurses. *Crit Care Nurs Clin North Am.* 2003;15:305-312.

4. O'Malley P, Trimble N, Browning M. Herbal therapies update: implications for the clinical nurse specialist. *Clin Nurse Spec.* 2002;16:173-177.

5. Tracy M, Lindquist R. Nursing's role in CAT use in critical care. *Crit Care Nurs Clin North Am.* 2003;15: 289-294.

6. Lindquist R, Tracy M, Savik K. Personal use of complementary and alternative therapies by critical care nurses. *Crit Care Nurs Clin North Am.* 2003;15:393-399.

7. Dossey BM, Keegan L, Guzzetta C. *Holistic Nursing: A Handbook for Practice.* 3rd ed. Sudbury, Mass: Jones & Bartlett Publishing; 2004.

8. Selye H. History of the stress concept. In: Goldberger L, ed. *Handbook of Stress: Theoretical and Clinical Aspects.* 2nd ed. New York, NY: The Free Press; 1993:7-17.

ASSOCIATIONS, ORGANIZATIONS, DATABASES, AND INTERNET RESOURCES FOR COMPLEMENTARY AND ALTERNATIVE MEDICINE

Internet Resources
- www.nccam.nih.gov
- www.altmedicine.com
- www.healthy.net
- www.womentowomen.com
- www.alternative-medicine-info.com
- www.holistic-online.com
- www.clinicaltrials.gov

Databases
- The Cochrane Library
- Traditional Chinese Medicine Database System
- CISCOM Database (Centralized Information Service for Complementary Medicine)

- MANTIS (Manual (Alternative and Natural Therapy Index)
- MicroMedex Complementary & Alternative Medicine Research Using Medline
- CAM on PubMed

Associations and Organizations
- Acupuncture and Oriental Medicine Alliance
- American Association for Health Freedom (formerly the Preventive Medical Association)
- American Botanical Council
- American Holistic Medical Association
- American Holistic Nursing Association
- American Massage Therapy Association
- Homeopathic Medical Association
- International Chiropractic Association
- National Center for Homeopathy

CLINICAL RECOMMENDATIONS

The rating scale for the Level of Recommendation ranges from I to VI, with levels indicated as follows: I, manufacturer's recommendations only; II, theory based, no research data to support recommendations; recommendations from expert consensus group may exist; III, laboratory data only, no clinical data to support recommendations; IV, limited clinical studies to support recommendations; V, clinical studies in more than 1 or 2 different populations and situations to support recommendations; VI, clinical studies in a variety of patient populations and situations to support recommendations.

Sphere of Influence	Recommendations	Rationale for Recommendation	Level of Recommendation	Supporting References	Comments
General CAM therapies recommended for patients and staff members	Patients: CAM therapies are useful during: • Painful procedures • Decreased ability to sleep • For manifestations of pain and anxiety such as anger, depression, agitation, disorientation, increased heart rate and respiratory rate, increased oxygen consumption, unexplained nausea and vomiting, diarrhea, and involuntary shaking Staff: CAM therapies are useful for: • Decreased ability to sleep • Inability to concentrate • Muscle tension and perceived increase in anxiety • Manifestations of anxiety such as anger, panic feelings, constant fatigue, diarrhea, and hyperventilation.	In both patients and staff members, use of alternative therapies can provide a sense of control over the situation, reduce adverse physiological effects of sleep deprivation, reduce anxiety and its manifestations, and reduce the physiological effects of the stress response. Alternative therapies also contribute to physical healing in patients and reduce the number of stress-related illnesses in staff members.	IV: Limited clinical studies to support recommendations	Annotated Bib: 1 References: 10, 12, 13 Suggested Readings: 1, 3, 5, 7	
Imagery	Imagery is useful for patients and staff in the following situations: Patients: • Painful or stressful procedures such as dressing changes, insertion or removal of tubes and suctioning • Anxiety Staff: • To improve performance in learning new skills • To decrease anxiety	Imagery helps persons improve their performance and control their responses to stressful situations. It is often used with relaxation to foster better visualization of images.	V. Clinical studies in more than 1 or 2 different populations or situations	Annotated Bib: 2, 3 References: 12, 13, 14, 21	

Sphere of Influence	Recommendations	Rationale for Recommendation	Level of Recommendation	Supporting References	Comments
Imagery (*cont.*)	*Application* *Patients* To implement imagery with a patient, do the following: 1. Gain the confidence of the patient so that he or she can relax and feel secure with you as a guide. 2. Close the curtains around the patient or use other measures to ensure privacy and prevent disturbances during the imagery experience. 3. Begin the session by taking the patient through deep breathing and relaxation exercises. 4. Continue the session by having the patient focus on a mental image of the specific area that requires health. 5. Verbally assist the patient to visualize a specific healing process that you describe. 6. Close the session with affirmations that the body will remember this experience and continue the healing process. 7. Follow-up with repeat versions of the exercises at periodic intervals. *Staff* To use imagery for staff members, do the following: 1. Begin a focus group of interested staff members who want to explore how the use of imagery can help in routine stress management. 2. Serve as a guide for the group or seek an external expert who can lead the staff in periodic guided imagery sessions.				

Sphere of Influence	Recommendations	Rationale for Recommendation	Level of Recommendation	Supporting References	Comments
Massage	Massage is indicated for patients and staff members with the following conditions: *Patients* • Generalized discomfort • Specific pain circumstances such as back pain or muscle pain *Staff* • Increased tension • Back, neck or foot pain • Fatigue *Application* Massage should be offered to all patients. To implement massage therapy in patients, do the following: 1. Inform the patient that his or her privacy will be ensured. 2. Procure massage lotion or oil and drape the patient. Place a bath towel at the patient's side. 3. Use the four primary back care strokes (see Appendix 5A).	A piece of skin the size of a quarter contains more than 3 million cells, 12 feet (3.6 m) of nerves, 100 sweat glands, 50 nerve endings, and 3 feet (0.9 m) of blood vessels. According to estimates, the skin has approximately 50 receptors per 100 cm2, a total of 900,000 sensory receptors. From this perspective, the skin is a giant communication system that, through the sense of touch, brings messages from the external environment to the attention of the internal environment: the body and mind.	VI: Clinical studies in a variety of populations and situations	Other References: 43-50	See Appendix 5A for Application guidelines
Relaxation	*Indications* Relaxation therapy is indicated for patients and staff members for the following conditions or situations: *Patients* • After painful or stressful procedures. • Sleep deprivation • Nausea and vomiting • Increased general anxiety *Staff* • When anxiety is increased, such as before the beginning of a shift or at the end of a shift.	General relaxation techniques work as a vehicle to initiate the relaxation response. Relaxation helps lower blood pressure, heart rate, and respiratory rate. Relaxation also quiets the mind, focuses thinking, and develops self-awareness.	V. Clinical studies in more than 1 or 2 different populations or situations	Annotated Bib: 5 References: 52 Other References: 51-53	The most common forms of relaxation therapy helpful in the acute and critical care environments are as follows: 1. Breathing exercises 2. Autogenics, or the teaching of self-generated positive inner phrases such as, "My breathing is calm and relaxed." 3. General relaxation response 4. Massage therapy 5. Body scanning that focuses on detecting areas of tension.

Sphere of Influence	Recommendations	Rationale for Recommendation	Level of Recommendation	Supporting References	Comments
Relaxation (*cont.*)	*Staff (cont.)* • After intense emergencies to reduce the stress response • Insomnia *Application* The following may be included in implementing relaxation in patients or staff members: • Assess to determine the most appropriate form of relaxation therapy for the situation. • Gain the confidence of the participant(s) in you as a guide by describing the process and the benefits that can be achieved. • Consider combining relaxation techniques with music and imagery techniques. • Establish an environment that promotes relaxation and privacy. • Use an appropriate script for obtaining the best relaxation response. • Apply massage strokes as appropriate to reduce tension and anxiety (see Appendix 5A).				Two basic steps are used to elicit the relaxation response: (1) the repetition of a word, sound, prayer, thought, phrase, or muscular activity; and (2) the passive return to the repetition when other thoughts intrude.
Prayer	*Indications* Prayer is recommended for both patients and staff to: • Relieve stress, anxiety, and tension • Combat depression • Assist in coping with fear of the unknown, pain • Experience a sense of control, activism in the healing process • Align one's personal will with the will of a higher power • Seek healing, direction, and peacefulness	Spiritual and religious practices, including prayer, are generally associated with positive impact on the perception of wellness and decreased morbidity and mortality. Practitioners of prayer obviously believe in its relevance and impact on health. Despite the conflicting opinions and research findings regarding the effectiveness of prayer, it is the most widely practiced of the CAM practices.	V. Clinical studies in more than 1 or 2 populations or situations	Annotated Bib: 2, 3 References: 22-31, 34-36, 38-41 Other References: 1-26	

Sphere of Influence	Recommendations	Rationale for Recommendation	Level of Recommendation	Supporting References	Comments
Biologically Based Practices	• Standardized products should be used. • Products with multiple herbs should be avoided. • All patients should be asked about herbal use and potential drug-herb, herb-herb interactions.	Herbals include processed and unprocessed parts of plants, extracts, and essential oils. May also include or be combined with vitamins, minerals, and animal products. Herbals have been used for centuries, but there is limited evidence for efficacy in vast majority of herbal products. Standardization process creates more consistent products. Multiple herbals in one product may lead to increased risk for toxicity. There are known interactions between herbs and drugs.	IV. Limited studies to support recommendations	Annotated Bib: 4 References: 7, 44, 48, 50 Suggested Readings: 2, 3 Other References: 27-42	

ANNOTATED BIBLIOGRAPHY

The citations in this bibliography are divided into four sections: stress management, spirituality and prayer, biologically based practices, and mind-body practices.

Stress Management

1. **Edwards D, Burnard P. Integrative literature reviews and meta-analyses: a systematic review of stress and stress management interventions for mental health nurses.** *J Adv Nurs.* 2003; 42(2):169-200.

Study Sample

176 papers, of which 70 met the inclusion criteria. Following completion of the initial review, 7 additional studies were reviewed and included in the published article. Studies included United Kingdom and non-United Kingdom research.

Study Procedures

A systematic review of research published between 1966 and 2000 was done. Inclusion criteria were publications in English, specific identification of participants as mental health nurses, and studies of effectiveness of stress management interventions.

Key Findings

The systematic review revealed that a great deal of knowledge exists regarding sources of stress at work and measurement of stress and outcome indicators. However, there was a lack of translation and application of this knowledge into practice.

Strengths and Weaknesses

Review included English-only studies. Methodological flaws in many of the reviewed studies reduced the rigor of some included studies.

Spirituality and Prayer

2. **Helm H, Hays J, Flint E, Koenig H, Blazer D. Does private religious activity prolong survival? A six-year follow-up study of 3,851 older adults.** *J Gerontol A Biol Sci Med Sci.* 2000 Jul;55(7): M400-5.

Study Sample

The probability sample consisted of 3851 elderly community-dwelling adults living in North Carolina.

Comparison Studied

The study used a prospective cohort design to determine if level of participation in private religious activities such as prayer, meditation, church attendance, use of religious media, or Bible study, as assessed by self-report at baseline, affected a wide variety of sociodemographic and health variables.

Study Procedures

The sample was a population-based, stratified random sample. Private religious activity was assessed by the question "How often do you spend time in private religious activities such as prayer, meditation, or Bible study?" Participants were placed in 1 of 5 groups based upon responses. Vital status was assessed through annual follow-up interviews and data abstracted from death certificates. Physical health variables included chronic conditions and inability to perform one or more activities of daily living (ADLs). If 2 blood pressures taken averaged greater than 140 systolic or more than 90 diastolic, a diagnosis of hypertension was included. Participants were asked to self-rate their health as good, fair, or poor. Presence of depression was assessed through use of the CES-D depression score, and negative life events, such as deaths of family members and divorce, were also surveyed. Finally, social connections and health practices were included. Baseline associations between private religious activity and all covariates were analyzed using the chi-square test. The association between private religious activity and survival was evaluated first, and then each of the covariates were added, using a Cox proportional hazards regression model. A dose-dependent and threshold effect was tested for. Four dummy variables were also constructed to test the benefit of increasing religious activity.

Key Findings

This study found that participation in nonorganizational religious activities, in those without impairment in the activities of daily living, had a protective effect against mortality. No such protective effect was demonstrated in participants who were already impaired in the activities of daily living. Females were more likely to be active in religious activities. Additionally, a report of lower religious activity was found in participants who were younger, Caucasian, and urban dwelling. Survival was significantly higher in the group with both reported religious activity and no impairment in ADL. This benefit persisted in this group after controlling for demographic, health, health practices, social support, and other religious practices. These results were expected based upon previous research.

Strengths and Weaknesses

Study strengths include a large sample size, longitudinal design, high response rate (80%), and control of extraneous variance through adjustment for multiple confounding variables. Weaknesses include a lack of specificity regarding types of prayer and devotional activities. Information regarding nutritional status and exercise was also missing.

3. Astin J, Harkness E, Ernst E. The efficacy of "distant healing": a systematic review of randomized trials. *Ann Int Med.* 2000;132:903-910.

Study Sample

Studies chosen for the systematic review were identified by an electronic search of MEDLINE, PsychLIT, MBASE, CISCOM, and Cochrane Library databases for the topics of distant healing, prayer, mental healing, therapeutic touch, or spiritual healing. Study inclusion criteria were randomization, placebo or other adequate control, clinical instead of experimental research, human subjects, and publication in refereed journals. Of the 23 studies that met inclusion criteria 5 were studies of prayer, 11 were therapeutic touch, 7 involved nonprayer forms of distant healing.

Study Procedures

Two investigators worked independently to extract data regarding study design, sampling procedures and sample size, types of interventions and controls, direction of effect, and descriptions of outcomes. A total of 23 trials with a collective sample of 2774 subjects met the inclusion criteria. Heterogeneity prevented a formal meta-analysis.

Key Findings

Of the 23 studies, 13 (57%) yielded statistically significant treatment effects, 9 showed no effect over control interventions, and 1 showed a negative effect.

Strengths and Weaknesses

Methodological weaknesses of the included studies made it difficult to draw definitive conclusions regarding the efficacy of distant healing. Given that 57% of the studies showed a positive treatment effect, the study of distant healing merits continued study.

Biologically Based Practices

4. Pittler MH, Ernst E. Kava extract for treating anxiety. Cochrane Database of Systematic Reviews. December 2003.

Study Sample

Eleven trials with a total of 645 participants met the inclusion criteria. Selection criteria included randomized, controlled trials or conducted placebo-controlled and double-blind studies. Trials using oral preparations containing kava extract as the only component were considered. Studies using kava as one of several components were excluded. Six trials used the Hamilton Anxiety scale as a common outcome measure. Two reviewers independently reviewed all included studies. Disagreements were resolved through discussion.

Study Procedures

Data were extracted systematically according to patient characteristics, interventions, and results. Methodological quality was assessed using the Jadad scoring system.

Key Findings

Compared with placebo, kava extract appears to be effective in the treatment of symptoms associated with anxiety. Data available demonstrated relative safety for short-term use of kava (1-24 weeks). Adverse events were mild, transient, and infrequent.

Strengths and Weaknesses

Citation tracking proved to be difficult and therefore possibly limited the completeness of this review.

Mind-Body Practices

5. Huntley A, White AR, Ernst E. Relaxation therapies for asthma: a systematic review. *Thorax.* 2002:57:127-131.

Study Sample

Fifteen trials were identified. Nine trials appropriately compared the treatment group with the control group.

Study Procedures

Four independent literature searches were performed using mainline databases. Only RCTs were included. There was no limitation on languages included. Two independent reviewers assessed the studies.

Key Findings

There is a lack of evidence for the efficacy of relaxation therapies for the management of asthma. Muscular relaxation techniques showed modest improvement of lung function, but there was no other evidence for other relaxation techniques.

Strengths and Weaknesses

A lack of rigor and methodological weaknesses explains the lack of evidence for efficacy.

OTHER REFERENCES

Spirituality and Prayer

1. Ai A, Bolling S, Peterson C. The use of prayer by coronary artery bypass patients. *Int J for Psychol Religion.* 2000;10(4):205-220.
2. Asser SM, Swan K. Child fatalities from religion-motivated medical neglect. *Pediatrics.* 1998;101:625-629.
3. Benson H. *Timeless Healing.* New York, NY: Fireside; 1996.
4. Byrd RC. Positive therapeutic effects of intercessory

prayer in a coronary care unit population. *Southern Med.* 1988;81:826-829.

5. Cavendish R, Konecny L, Kraynyak B, Lanza M. Nurses enhance performance through prayer. *Holistic Nurs Pract.* 2004;18(1):26-31.

6. Emblen J. Religion and spirituality defined according to current use in nursing literature. *J Profess Nurs.* 1992; 8(1):41-47.

7. Emblen J, Halstead L. Spiritual needs and interventions: comparing the views of patients, nurses, and chaplains. *Clin Nurse Special.* 1993;7:175-182.

8. Francis LJ. Denominational identity, church attendance, and drinking behavior among adults in England. *J Alcohol Drug Educ.* 1994;39:27-33.

9. Gorsuch, RL. Religious aspects of substance abuse and recovery. *J Soc Issues.* 1993;25:65-83.

10. Hutch RL, Burg MA, Naberhaus DS, Hellmich LK. The Spiritual Involvement and Beliefs Scale. *J Fam Pract.* 1998;46:476-486.

11. Kaczorowski JM. Spiritual well-being and anxiety in adults diagnosed with cancer. *Hospice J.* 1989;5:105-126.

12. King DE, Bushwick B. Beliefs and attitudes of hospital inpatients about faith healing and prayer. *Fam Pract.* 1994;39:349-352.

13. Koenig HG, Cohen HG, George LK, Hays JC, Larson DB, Blazer DG. Attendance at religious services, interleukin-6, and other biological parameters of immune function in older adults. *Int Psychiatry Med.* 1997;27:233-250.

14. Krebs K. The spiritual aspect of caring: an integral part of health and healing. *Nurs Admin Q.* 2001;25(3):55-60.

15. Landis BJ. Uncertainty, spiritual well-being and psychosocial adjustment to chronic illness. Issues *Ment Health Nurs.* 1996;27:217-231.

16. Marwick C. Should physicians prescribe prayer for health? Spiritual aspects of well-being considered. *JAMA.* 1995;273:1561-1562.

17. Morris EL. The relationship of spirituality to coronary heart disease. *Alternative Ther Health Med.* 2001;7(5): 96-98.

18. Newberg A, Pourdehnad M, Alavi A, d'Aquili EG. Cerebral blood flow during meditative prayer: preliminary findings and methodological issues. *Percept Motor Skills.* 97(2):625-630.

19. Oxman TE, Freeman DH, Mannheimer ED. Lack of social participation or religious strength and comfort as risk factors after cardiac surgery in the elderly. *Psychosom Med.* 1995;57:5-15.

20. Pargament KI. *Theory, Research, Practice. The Psychology of Religion and Coping.* New York, NY: Guilford; 1997.

21. Pressman P. Religious belief, depression and ambulation status in elderly women with broken hips. *Am J Psychiatry.* 1990;147:758-760.

22. Roberts L, Ahmed I, Hall S. Intercessory prayer for the alleviation of ill health. 2003. Available at: http://www.cochrane.org/reviews/en/ab000368.html. Accessed November 8, 2006.

23. Sherwood GD. The power of nurse-client encounters: interpreting spiritual themes. *J Holistic Nurs.* 2000; 18(2):159-175.

24. Vandenbrouke JP. Decreased mortality among contemplative monks in the Netherlands. *Am J Epidemiol.* 1996; 141(771-775).

25. Winslow GR, Winslow BW. Examining the ethics of praying with patients. *Holistic Nurs Pract.* 17:170-177.

26. Zinnbauer BJ, Pargament KL, Cowell BJ, Rye M, Scott AB. Religion and spirituality: unfuzzing the fuzzy. *J Sci Stud Religion.* 1997;38:412-423.

Biologicals

27. Agency for Healthcare Research and Quality. *AHRQ Issues New Report on the Safety and Effectiveness of Melatonin Supplements.* Rockville, Md: AHRQ; 2004.

28. Barnes P, Powell-Griner E, McFann K, Nahin R. Complementary and alternative medicine use among adults: United States, 2002. Available at: http:nccam.nih.gov/news/report.pdf. Accessed November 8, 2006.

29. Bent S, Ko R. Commonly used herbal medicines in the United States: a review. *Am J Med.* 2004;116:478-485.

30. Cairney S, Maruff P, Clough AR. The neurobehavioral effects of kava. *Aust N Z J Psychiatry.* 2002;36(5):657-662.

31. Davidson RJ, Kabat-Zinn J, Schumacher J, et al. Alterations in brain and immune function produced by mindfulness meditation. *Psychosom Med.* 2003;65(4):564-570.

32. DeLeo V, La Marca A, Morgante G, Lanzetta D, Floria P, Petraglia F. Evaluation of combining kava extract with hormone replacement therapy in the treatment of postmenopausal anxiety. *Maturitas.* 2001;39(2):185-188.

33. Greenburg PE, Sisitsky T, Kessler RC, Finkelstein SN, Berndt ER, Davidson JR. The economic burden of anxiety disorders in the 1990s. *J Clin Psychiatry.* 1999;60: 427-435.

34. Harkey MR, Henderson GL, Gershwin ME, et al. Variability in commercial ginseng products: an analysis of 25 preparations. *Am J Clin Nutr.* 2001;73:1101-1106.

35. Harnack LJ, Rydell SA, Stang J. Prevalence of use of herbal products by adults in the Minneapolis/St Paul, Minn, metropolitan area. *Mayo Clin Proc.* 2001;76: 688-694.

36. Kim HL, Streltzer J, Goebert D. St. John's wort for depression: a meta-analysis of well-defined clinical trials. *J Nerv Ment Dis.* 1999;187:532-538.

37. Lehman E, Klieser E, Klimke A, Krach H, Spatz R. The efficacy of cavain in patients suffering from anxiety. *Pharmacopsychiatry.* 1989;22(6):258-262.

38. Pittler MH, Ernst E. Kava extract for treating anxiety. *Cochrane Database Syst Rev.* 2003;(1):CD003383.

39. Rotblatt M, Ziment I. *Evidence-based Herbal Medicine.* Philadelphia, Penn: Hanley & Belfus Inc; 2002.

40. Shelton RC, Keller MB, Gelenberg A, et al. Effectiveness of St. John's wort in major depression (Cochrane Review): a randomized controlled trial. *JAMA.* 2001 285:1978-1986.

41. Singh NN, Ellis CR, Sharp I, Eakin K, Best AM, Singh YN. A double-blind, placebo-controlled study of the effects of kava on daily stress and anxiety in adults. *Alternative Ther.* 1998;4:97-98.

42. US Food and Drug Administration, Center for Food Safety and Applied Nutrition. *Dietary Supplements: Questions and Answers.* Washington, DC: USDA; 2001.

Massage

43. Wells-Federman CL, Stuart EM, Deckro JP, Mandle CL, Baim M, Medick C. The body-mind connection: the psychophysiology of many traditional nursing interventions. *Clin Nurse Spec.* 1995 Jan;9(1):59-66.

44. Hill CF. Massage in intensive care nursing: a literature review. *Compl Ther Med.* 1995;3:100-104.

45. Kirshbaum M. Using message in the relief of lymphodema. *Prof Nurse.* 1996;11:230-232.

46. Zuberbueler E. Complementary therapies in terminal care. Massage therapy: an added dimension in terminal care. *Am J Hospice Palliative Care.* 1996;13(2):50.

47. Wanning T. Healing and the mind/body arts: massage, acupuncture, yoga, tai chi. and Feldenkrais. *AAOHN J.* 1993;41:349-351.

48. Hill CF. Is massage beneficial to critically ill patients in intensive care units? A critical review. *Intensive Crit Care Nurs.* 1993;9:116-121.

49. White J. Touching with intent: therapeutic massage. *Holist Nurs Pract.* 1988;2:63-67.

50. Snyder M. Interventions for decreasing agitation behaviors in persons with dementia. *J Gerontol Nurs.* 1995; 21:34-40.

Relaxation

51. Syrjala K. Relaxation and imagery and cognitive behavioral training reduce pain during cancer treatment: a controlled clinical trial. *Pain.* 1995;2:160,190.

52. Sloman R. Relaxation and the relief of cancer pain. *Nurs Clin North Am.* 1995;4:667,700.

53. Mandle CL, Jacobs SC, Arcari PM, Domar AD. The efficacy of relaxation response interventions with adult patients: a review of the literature. *J Cardiovasc Nurs.* 1996;10(3):4,26.

Giving a Back Massage

Ask the patient to lie flat on his or her abdomen, if possible. Otherwise, have the patient lie on his or her side. Stand beside the patient, and place your hands on the patient's back for a moment as you begin contact. Your hands should contain warmed lotion or oil, and the patient should be emotionally and physically prepared for the back massage.

Once you begin the procedure, keep at least one hand on the patient's body at all times. The massage consists of four basic strokes:

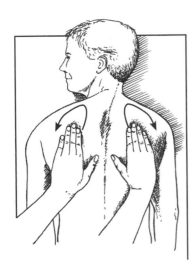

Figure 5A-1

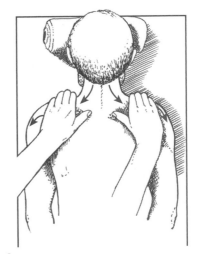

Figure 5A-2

1. *Effleurage* (Figure 5A-1): Slow upward motions along the length of the back from the waist to the shoulders. Begin by moving your hands slowly up the patient's back alongside the spine all the way to the sides of the neck. Then separate your hands, and move them across the shoulders and then down along the side of the back, returning to the waist. Repeat this stroke several times.

2. *Pétrissage* (Figure 5A-2): A kneading technique done alongside the length of the back, concentrating on the shoulders from the neck to the arms. Use medium to moderate pressure, and observe the patient for any indication of pain or pleasure. Ask the patient to give you feedback if no response is forthcoming without solicitation. Find an area or areas that seem to be the most soothing and spend more time there.

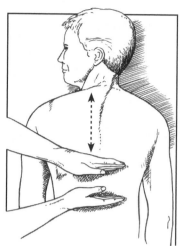

Figure 5A-3

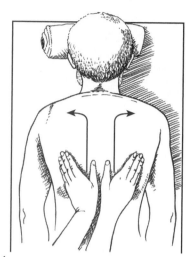

Figure 5A-4

3. *Tapotement* (Figure 5A-3): A tapping or chopping stroke done with the side edge of the hand moving from the waist to the shoulders along the flat of the back. This stroke is stimulating and may not be appropriate for critically ill patients. Use this stroke with discretion.

4. *Effleurage* (Figure 5A-4): Slow soothing motions done to conclude the massage. This stroke is a repeat of the one used to begin the massage. Begin with medium pressure, and gradually decrease it to a light touch. Remove your hands from the patient's body, and immediately cover the patient to ensure warmth. Allow the patient to rest or sleep before initiating any other therapy.

Pain Management

Richard B. Arbour, RN, MSN, CCRN, CNRN

Pain Management

CASE STUDY

R.B., a 34-year-old man, was evaluated in the emergency department at 11:00 AM following a fall down 5 steps in his home. On initial assessment and triage he was found to have extreme pain and tenderness distally in his left upper extremity involving the wrist and lower forearm. He described his pain as a score of 10 on a scale of 0-10 where 10 represents the worst pain possible. The pain became significantly more intense with any movement or palpation. This made it very difficult to position the extremity for diagnostic radiographic studies. Intravenous (IV) access was established with an 18-gauge catheter, and R.B. received 0.9% saline at 50 cc/hour. Analgesia was provided with IV morphine sulfate beginning with a 2 mg bolus and titrated as needed. Frequent bolus doses were given to keep R.B. comfortable, with a pain score goal of 1/10. This required a cumulative dosage of 24 mg over 1 and 1.5 hours.

Vital signs and oxygen saturation were initially stable. Two hours following initial evaluation and treatment, and pending definitive evaluation of his orthopedic injury, R.B. became progressively short of breath, desaturated to an oxygen saturation of 85% (from 97%) on room air and remained hypoxemic following application of supplemental oxygen by face mask at 50%. R.B. became less responsive over the ensuing 15 minutes and his breathing was supported with manual ventilation using a bag-valve-mask system and 100% oxygen pending endotracheal intubation and controlled ventilation. An additional IV access was obtained with an 18-gauge catheter. Immediately prior to endotracheal intubation R.B. received propofol 25 mg IV bolus for sedation to facilitate endotracheal intubation. After placing/securing the airway and verifying proper endotracheal tube placement by clinical assessment and radiographically, R.B.

was then admitted to the medical intensive care unit (MICU) for further evaluation and treatment of pulmonary compromise with appropriate orthopedic consultation to manage his left upper extremity injury.

R.B. had a past medical history significant for chronic obstructive pulmonary disease (COPD), heavy smoking (2 packs per day for 15 years) and heavy alcohol (ETOH) use, consuming approximately six 12-ounce cans of beer per day. Due to a prior back injury, R.B. suffered from chronic, moderately severe pain for which he was prescribed and took 2 tablets of percocet 4 times daily. He had a history of anxiety which was treated with lorazepam 1 mg by mouth twice daily. From an automobile accident 7 years ago R.B. suffered a mild chest wall contusion from which he had fully recovered. Previous surgeries included an appendectomy 12 years prior to admission. He weighed 77 kg (approximately 169 lb) and was 179 cm (70 inches) tall.

In the MICU, his initial vital signs were as follows: heart rate, 98 beats per minute; blood pressure, 154/76 mm Hg; mean arterial pressure, 102 mm Hg; respirations, 24-28 breaths per minute, assisting the ventilator; arterial oxygen saturation is 96% on fraction of inspired oxygen (FIO_2), 0.50, and body temperature, 36.5°C (97.8°F). Neurologically R.B. was responsive to voice and followed simple commands. He was able to communicate by nodding his head appropriately in response to questions and had intact cranial nerves. His protective reflexes were intact and he had a vigorous cough reflex during endotracheal suctioning. He was able to move all his extremities. He had full strength in both legs and the right arm. Movement was significantly restricted in his left arm due to pain from his orthopedic injury. First and second heart sounds were audible on auscultation without murmurs, rubs, or gallops, and ECG monitoring showed normal sinus rhythm without ectopy. The skin was warm and dry, pulses were 3+ in all extremities with capillary refill time of less than 3 seconds. The mucous membranes were pink and moist, and he had no peripheral edema. Complete blood count and chemistry test results were within normal limits.

Breath sounds were clear but decreased, with occasional rhonchi that resolved following endotracheal suctioning. Endotracheal aspirate consisted of moderate amounts of moderately thick white secretions. Chest wall excursion was not restricted during controlled ventilation; however, even minimal movement to reposition R.B. was exquisitely painful due to the orthopedic injury. Even when lying quietly, R.B. was increasingly anxious, which appeared to increase his pain perception.

R.B. was having episodes of increasingly severe anxiety and restlessness compounded by tracheal intubation, controlled ventilation, pain due to a potentially unstable fracture involving his left upper extremity, preexisting back pain, and feelings of loss of control being a patient in a critical care unit. Upon even minimal movement of the affected extremity R.B. exhibited significant nonverbal pain behaviors including severe grimacing, wincing, and general muscle rigidity.

Pain/Anxiety Status

There were clearly multiple components to R.B.'s pain, anxiety, and agitation:

- He had a preexisting anxiety disorder. For this comorbidity R.B. was treated with lorazepam 2 mg IV bolus every 4 hours. The IV lorazepam was also an effective prophylaxis for potential ETOH withdrawal while in the intensive care unit.
- He had baseline back pain as well as being at risk of narcotic withdrawal syndrome due to his long-term opioid use. This was addressed by administration of morphine sulfate in divided doses up to 12 mg over a 1-hour period maintaining adequate analgesia for 2 hours. At this time R.B. was rebolused with morphine sulfate 8 mg IV followed by the start of a morphine sulfate infusion at 6 mg per hour. This resulted in relief of R.B.'s back pain while he remained responsive to stimulation. Coordination between bolus and infusion dosing of morphine was important to more rapidly attain therapeutic plasma concentrations of the analgesic. The coordinated use of bolus and infusion dosing also will maintain a steady level of analgesia while avoiding peaks and troughs in analgesia with resultant oversedation or undertreatment of pain leading to breakthrough pain.
- There was a risk of nicotine withdrawal in the intensive care unit due to R.B.'s history of heavy smoking. This was addressed by prescribing a high-dose nicotine transdermal system at a delivered dose of 21 mg per day.
- R.B. was uncomfortable from being intubated and on controlled ventilation with resultant dyssynchrony between the ventilator and his own respiratory cycle. This was addressed by titration of ventilator settings including initiation of continuous positive airway pressure (CPAP) and pressure support ventilation (PSV). These settings were quickly titrated to R.B.'s comfort and ventilator synchrony. These interventions gave R.B. significantly better control over the rate, depth, and pattern of his respiratory cycle. Although R.B. still experienced discomfort from his artificial airway, he was no longer dyssynchronous with controlled ventilation, had far fewer surges in intrathoracic pressure with resultant pain and agitation, and was subjectively far more comfortable and accepting of care.
- The acute pain associated with his orthopedic injury, and how exquisitely sensitive his left wrist and forearm were to even minimal stimulation, produced severe breakthrough pain. This pain was exhibited by nonverbal indications such as increased muscle/motor tension, grimacing, changes in rate and pattern of respiratory cycle, as well as furrowing of his brow and diaphoresis. This issue was of particular concern for R.B. because it interfered with optimal positioning of the affected extremity for definitive radiographic diagnosis. It would also make reduction/stabilization of the fracture prior to any potential surgical intervention more difficult. This pain was relieved by IV bolus dosing with fentanyl citrate (250 µg over 20 minutes) and IV lorazepam (5 mg over 25 minutes) prior to manipulation of the affected extremity. IV fentanyl was administered preemptively to avoid as much as possible initiating the cycle of pain, anxiety, and agitation. Opioid analgesia was administered concurrently with IV lorazepam for multiple reasons. First, anxiety was a preexisting component of R.B.'s clinical issues, and pain will increase anxiety, which then can increase pain perception in a cyclical phenomenon. Second, the synergistic interactions between the 2 classes of central nervous system (CNS) depressants enabled lower doses from both drug classes and facilitates recovery from procedural sedation. Having received opioid analgesia and benzodiazepine sedation concurrently for manipulation of the affected extremity during radiographic studies, R.B. tolerated the procedure well, with minimal discomfort based on assessment of nonverbal pain behaviors.

With his condition stabilized pending preparations for open reduction internal fixation (ORIF) of the fractures, lung function improved and planning began for weaning from ventilation. Given that R.B. was scheduled for surgery within the next 24 hours, aggressive weaning proceeding to extubation was not the most practical option. His salient issues including risk of withdrawal (opioid, benzodiazepine, ETOH, and nicotine) were effectively addressed. Cardiopulmonary issues including hemodynamic stability and control of bronchospasm/COPD were addressed with administration of fluid volume, titration of ventilator settings/F_{IO_2}, and administration of bronchodilators. The plan was to aggressively wean and extubate as quickly as possible following surgery.

Of particular concern was the need for effective opioid analgesia postoperatively. Given his history of COPD and opioid tolerance, high-dose opioids usually given to provide optimal analgesia in the postoperative period were considered a possible risk factor for prolonged recovery, delayed weaning from controlled ventilation, and increased length of stay (LOS) in the MICU for R.B. For these reasons, the anesthesia provider was consulted preoperatively about using an axillary block for postoperative analgesia. R.B. had no comorbidities such as nutrition depletion, thrombocytopenia, or coagulopathy as contraindications to this type of invasive analgesia.

At 8:00 AM the following morning, R.B. was transported to the OR for ORIF. The procedure took approximately 2.5 hours and, as planned, the anesthesiologist utilized an axillary block for postoperative analgesia. Following recovery from anesthesia, and on return to the MICU, R.B. was comfortable with the analgesia provided by the axillary block. It reduced the need for additional opioid analgesia, although such was still required for preexisting back pain. He also continued to receive IV lorazepam to manage anxiety and prevent ETOH withdrawal syndrome. Neither intervention resulted in significant cardiopulmonary depression or delayed the weaning process.

Soon after returning to the MICU, aggressive weaning from controlled ventilation was pursued. R.B. was awake, interactive, and accepting of care, when asked if he was in pain he responded by shaking his head "no." He did not demonstrate nonverbal indications of pain. Extubation proceeded smoothly, and R.B. continued to recover.

The next day (postoperative day 1) oral agents were instituted to replace his IV sedation and analgesia. For R.B.'s preexisting back pain, percocet, 2 tablets every 4 hours, was administered to maintain steady-state analgesia. Following the initial dose, his morphine infusion was titrated down and ultimately off as determined by his analgesia needs. For R.B.'s preexisting anxiety, and risk of ETOH withdrawal, lorazepam 2 mg by mouth was administered every 4 hours. Transdermal nicotine was continued to prevent nicotine withdrawal and followed up with counseling services and a smoking cessation program. These interventions produced the clinical end point of an awake, interactive patient who was not experiencing sedation as a side effect of medications. Postoperative pain (breakthrough) was managed with IV morphine 5 mg and titrated to comfort with a goal of a pain score of 1/10. Stress ulcer prophylaxis was started with pantoprazole (protonix) 40 mg, every 12 hours. Deep vein thrombosis (DVT) prophylaxis began with heparin sodium 5000 units every 12 hours subcutaneously.

With successful weaning and extubation, adequate analgesia, and control of factors contributing to increased pain R.B. continued to improve and his condition remained stable. His vital signs were stable and he was oxygenating and ventilating well. R.B. stated that his preexisting back pain and pain at his operative site (left arm) was well controlled. He reported getting adequate sleep during the previous night, felt better, and was able to increase his activity level. Assessment of nonverbal cues to pain revealed no grimacing, tremors, muscle/motor tension, agitation, furrowed brow, diaphoresis, or eyes tightly closed. He was at his goal pain score of 1/10 most of the time.

On postoperative day 3 he complained of feeling "too sleepy" with a pain score of "0." On further investigation, it was noted that this feeling and score occurred immediately following a dose of IV morphine 5 mg for breakthrough pain at his surgical site. The dose of IV morphine was decreased to 2 mg IV, which produced no further sedation as a side effect and produced adequate analgesia. R.B.'s regularly scheduled opioid and benzodiazepine therapy was continued, and he continued to receive IV morphine 2 mg in bolus dosing for breakthrough pain.

GENERAL DESCRIPTION

Pain is widely and correctly viewed as among the major stressors and worst fears experienced by acutely and critically ill patients. This fear is greater in the setting of palliative care delivery in the acute or critical care setting. Pain is common in all age groups and is frequently seen as an initial or concurrent complaint during events precipitating admission to a critical care unit.[1] Pain experienced by acute and critically ill patients may include pain of short duration or acute episodes as well as more chronic or long-term pain states.[2] Short-term or acute pain may be caused by the pathophysiologic process, illness or injury, or may be from invasive procedures such as chest tube thoracostomy, endotracheal suctioning, or even positioning in bed.[3,4,5] Chronic or long-term pain may be caused by prolonged tissue injury from inflammatory processes, positioning, or pain produced by the existence and/or progression of metastatic disease.[2] Irrespective of whether pain is chronic or acute in origin there are multiple physiologic changes in response to the clinical state of pain that ultimately produce associated risks and complications.[1,2,6,7]

Virtually all of the physiologic consequences of pain are mediated through activation of the physiologic stress response.[1,2,6-8] Mobilization of the stress response is beneficial in the short-term to help maintain physiologic stability.[9] Over the long-term, mobilization of the stress response as seen with prolonged, unrelieved pain may cause increased morbidity related to multisystem consequences. Such consequences may include the following:

- Increased sympathetic outflow with increased global and myocardial oxygen consumption and metabolic rate
- Increased levels of circulating stress hormones such as catecholamines, cortisol, and glucagons

- Compromised immune response and hypercoagulable state
- Reduced gastrointestinal motility
- Psychosocial consequences including increased anxiety, agitation, and fear as well as the potential for development of an adversarial relationship with health care providers
- Protein catabolic state and negative nitrogen balance
- Fluid and electrolyte imbalances due to ADH secretion.[1,2,6,9,10-11]

These are compelling reasons for aggressive, comprehensive pain management in the critically ill patient. Beyond the provision of humane care and ensuring that the patient's rights for effective pain management are honored, attenuation of the potentially harmful physiologic consequences of unrelieved pain with the resulting risk reduction for the patient is crucial for healing.

Definition

Pain is defined as an "unpleasant sensory and emotional experience associated with actual or potential tissue damage, or described in terms of such damage."[12] Pain may also defined as an individualistic, physiologic, learned, and social response to a noxious stimuli.[13] Pain is by definition a subjective experience, and in a cognitively intact patient it is best described as "what the experiencing person says it is, existing whenever he says it does," and by definition should be taken very seriously.[14] Life experiences and background, emotional state, thought processes, and interpersonal environment all may influence an individual's pain response or the external expressions of pain.

Pain Physiology

There exist 2 main types of pain: nociceptive pain and neuropathic pain. Nociceptive pain begins with a process generally in the periphery such as a direct tissue injury or trauma. This tissue trauma causes the release of multiple substances or mediators from damaged areas. These include prostaglandins, bradykinin, serotonin, substance P, and histamine. When released in sufficient concentrations, these mediators stimulate nerve endings (nociceptors) within the periphery. Through a controlled membrane instability, sodium channels open, allowing entry of the sodium ion into the neuron, creating the action potential/nerve impulse. The nerve impulse is conducted through the sensory neuron toward the central nervous system (CNS). The specific pathways conducting the pain impulse to the CNS are the A-delta and C fibers, the distal endings of which are mostly comprised of nociceptors. The nerve fibers conduct the nociceptive information to the spinal cord, terminating in the dorsal horn of the spinal cord. Once the nerve fibers terminate in the dorsal horn of the spinal cord, neurotransmitters, specifically substance P, aspartate, glutamate, and adenosine triphosphate (ATP), are released to continue transmission of the pain impulse from the sensory neuron to the dorsal horn of the spinal cord. From the dorsal horn of the spinal cord,

transmission of the pain impulse continues upward to the brain through the ascending spinothalamic tracts. The next stop for the ascending pain impulses includes the brain stem and thalamus. The thalamus acts like a relay station, sending the pain impulses to other brain areas including the cerebral cortex where the conscious perception of pain occurs.

Depending on the severity of the original injury and subsequent tissue damage, a state of hyperalgesia, or markedly enhanced responsiveness to even minimal stimuli, causes acute pain. This may be primary or secondary in nature. Primary hyperalgesia occurs at the original site of tissue damage and is related to increased sensitivity of the nociceptors. Secondary hyperalgesia occurs in adjacent areas to the original injury and may result from sensitization of peripheral nociceptors or sensitization of central nociceptive neurons. [3-4,12,14,]

Pain Assessment

Pain perception and related behaviors may be affected by many factors including cultural background, education, prior experiences, ethnicity, locus of control, fatigue, sleep deprivation, anxiety, depression, regression, altered mental status, dementia, and delirium. Pain responses can be categorized as verbal, behavioral, and physiologic. Verbal responses are the gold standard for pain assessment. Their use however is limited to the cognitively intact patient who is able to effectively communicate. Behavioral responses to pain as guides to assessment and effectiveness of therapy are increasingly studied and validated in the professional literature.[5,15-16] Physiologic responses result from the activation of the sympathetic nervous system. These responses may cause multiple signs and symptoms commonly associated with mobilization of physiologic stress. In the setting of chronic pain, concurrent drug therapy, volume status, or disease state, symptoms of physiologic stress mobilization may not be reliable as indications of pain.[6,17] Moreover, a patient not exhibiting these physiologic changes may very well still be experiencing pain. It is very important to take a thorough pain history so that all health care team members are cognizant of the types of pain the patient may have as a normal baseline. This becomes important in assessing pain related to the current illness or injury.

Modulating Pain Transmission and Perception

The physiology of pain response and perception is a complex, multistep process. Each step in this process from tissue injury and peripheral nociception through the conscious perception of pain at the cerebral cortex is an opportunity for intervention involving modulating 1 or more parts of the overall pain pathway. Treatment options in managing nociceptive pain include centrally acting agents such as opioid analgesics, site-specific therapies such as nonsteroidal anti-inflammatory agents (NSAIDs), local and regional techniques, and using local anesthetic agents.[14]

Neuropathic pain is generally related to abnormal processing of sensory input that may occur following injury to the peripheral or central nervous system.[14] Neuropathic pain may be central or peripheral in origin. Central neuropathic pain may reflect injury to the dorsal horn of the spinal cord in which an otherwise benign stimulus may be interpreted as pain.[4] Peripheral neuropathic pain reflects injury to or abnormality within the peripheral nervous system. It may be felt by the patient along the distribution of 1 or more peripheral nerves.[4,14] In general, stimuli abnormally processed by the CNS may produce neuropathic pain. Treatment options in managing neuropathic pain include anticonvulsants, antiarrhythmics, and local anesthetics which are thought to be effective due to membrane-stabilizing effects and suppression of abnormal neuronal activity.[3,4,14] There are common neurochemical pathways between pain and depression, specifically serotonin and norepinephrine. Thus, additional options in managing neuropathic pain include antidepressants (tricyclic antidepressants) and selective-serotonin reuptake inhibitors (SSRIs).[18,19]

Site-Specific Therapy

Pain transmission may be modulated in multiple ways. One way is by therapeutic interventions that act at the site of injury. Agents such as nonsteroidal anti-inflammatory agents (NSAIDs), (ie, ketorolac tromethamine, ibuprofen, naproxen) appear to produce analgesia by 2 mechanisms: (1) inhibiting the COX-2 isoenzyme at the site of injury or inflammation with related reduction of prostaglandin synthesis; and (2) the anti-inflammatory effect of this class of drugs.[20-22] Pain as a consequence of orthopedic trauma in particular may especially benefit from therapy with NSAIDs.[23] Reduction in prostaglandin synthesis is important because prostaglandin sensitizes pain receptors to both chemical mediators as well as mechanical stimulation.

Centrally Acting Agents

Opioid analgesia has long been the mainstay of systemic or centrally acting analgesia for acute and critically ill patients. Opioids produce their clinical effects by binding to specific receptors within the brain, spinal cord, and peripheral tissues such as the GI tract.[6] There are 3 general types of opioid receptors (mu, kappa, and sigma). Of these, the mu receptor is primarily responsible for analgesia. The others (kappa and sigma) are responsible in varying degrees for mediating side effects of opioids such as dysphoria/delirium and hallucinations.[6,22,24] Table 6-1 illustrates select pharmacokinetics and dosing for opioid and reversal agents used in adult critical care.[6] Table 6-2 illustrates nursing considerations and side effects for selected sedative/narcotic agents used in critical care practice.[6]

Central Neuroaxis Techniques

Analgesia may be obtained through delivery of analgesic, anesthetic agents directly within the central neuroaxis such as occurs using epidural techniques. Epidural administration of opioid agonists works by binding of the opioid agonist to pre- and postsynaptic receptors within the substantia gelatinosa of the spinal cord. Motor and autonomic functions are unaffected. Local anesthetic administration is effective due to blockade of sodium channels and consequent blocking of neuronal impulses.[25,26]

Regional Techniques

An additional approach is through delivery of local anesthetic agents directly within a peripheral nerve innervating an injured extremity. One example of this technique may be seen with an axillary nerve block in an extremity following wrist fracture/ORIF in managing pain while minimizing systemic opioid dosing. There are multiple options for delivery of regional analgesia including intercostal, intrapleural, and brachial plexus techniques and intraperitoneal lavage. Administration of local anesthetic agents such as lidocaine or bupivicaine produces sodium channel blockade, thus preventing transmission of pain impulses. The central and regional deliveries of analgesia are invasive, and their use must be considered after careful weighing of their benefits in relation to the costs of their complications. If the benefits of minimizing systemic opioid dosing outweigh the potential complications, this an excellent analgesic technique.[27]

Pain in Special Populations of the Adult Critically Ill

Pain may be a near-universal experience for critically ill patients and is deserving of profound attention in all subgroups of patient demographics. Three patient subgroups of the adult population seen with increasing frequency in clinical practice that deserve additional attention include those patients receiving palliative care for a terminal phase of illness, those with a history of substance abuse, and elderly patients.

End-of-Life Situations

Despite much education in recent years as well as availability of advance directive options, an untold number of patients die annually in critical care units.[28] Causes of pain in this stage of illness and delivery of care may involve progression of metastatic disease, nerve damage, side effects of treatment, invasive devices, or preexisting tissue damage.[29] In these situations patients and their families must be assured that pain can and will be relieved. There are multiple options for analgesia including but not limited to increasing dosage or potency of opioid agents utilized.[29] Education should be provided to the family and patient as appropriate regarding the concept of double effect. This means that interventions to relieve pain in terminal care settings should be provided even when those interventions entail risk of hastening death.[30] In these situations death represents a natural and expected event in the progression of illness or injury that the clinician cannot alter. Aggressive relief of pain and suffering related to disease progression and/or the dying process is well within clinician control.[51] For example, severe pain may still exist following removal of an endotracheal tube after a family decides to withdraw curative aggressive treatment. In this

Table 6-1 Pharmacokinetics of Selected Sedatives and Analgesics and Their Reversal Agents Used in Critical Care of Adults

Agent	Intravenous dose	Distribution half-life, minutes	Elimination half-life (with metabolites), hours	Active metabolite	% Protein binding	Time of onset, minutes	Duration of action (with metabolites)	Average daily dose, milligrams	Average cost, US$
Benzodiazepines									
Lorazepam	0.25-2.0 mg	3	10-20	No	85-91	20-40	2-6 hours	65	180
Midazolam	0.02-0.08 mg/kg	1-2	1.0-12.3	Yes	95	1-5	1-6 hours	225	355
Diazepam	0.1 mg/kg (slow)	1-2	20-80	Yes	98-99	1-5	2-6 hours	50	18
Nonbenzodiazepine sedatives									
Propofol	5-50 µg/kg per minute (0.3-3.0 mg/kg per hour; some patients may need higher doses)	2-4.1	1-8.1	No	98	<1	3-8 minutes	3000	210
Neuroleptic									
Haloperidol	1-5 mg (initial)	3-19	12-22	Yes	92	<10	2-6 hours	30	40
Narcotics									
Morphine	2-10 mg	10-20	1.7-4.5	Yes	36	2-3	4-5 hours	100	5
Fentanyl	50-100 µg	10-30	2-4	No	84	1-2	30-60 minutes	4	55
Meperidine	0.5-1.5 mg/kg	4-11	3-8	Yes	58	1-2	2-4 hours	500	5
Hydromorphone	10-30 µg/kg	Limited information available	2.5-3.3	Yes	71	10-15	2-3 hours	25	7
Remifentanil	0.1 µg/kg per minute	0.75-1.0	0.33	Negligible	70	0.5-1.0	5-10 minutes	21	240
Reversal agents									
Naloxone	3-30 µg/kg	<5	1.4	No	30	<1	1-2 hours	70	180
Nalmefene	0.5-1.0 mg	<5	8.6	No	45	<3	8-10 hours	4.5	100
Flumazenil	3-45 µg/kg	Limited information available	0.85-1.0	No	50	<3	30-60 minutes	12	575

* Parameters such as dosages should be used as guidelines. All decisions on dosing should be based on a complete assessment. Treatment should be started with lower doses, and doses should be increased incrementally until the desired clinical end point is achieved. Average daily costs are based on wholesale prices; specific costs to institutions may vary.

Reprinted with permission.[6p43-44]

Table 6-2   Nursing Considerations and Side Effects of Selected Sedatives and Narcotics

Agent/class	Clinical actions	Side effects	Nursing considerations
Benzodiazepines			
Midazolam	Anxiolysis, amnesia, hypnosis	Hypotension Respiratory depression Paradoxical agitation	Increase doses slowly by increments with titration. Monitor blood pressure and respiratory status. Administer fluids as indicated. Slowly wean from drug after prolonged therapy.
Diazepam	Anxiolysis, amnesia, hypnosis	Hypotension Respiratory depression Paradoxical agitation	Increase doses slowly by increments with titration. Monitor blood pressure and respiratory status. Administer fluids as indicated. Slowly wean from drug after prolonged therapy.
Lorazepam	Anxiolysis, amnesia, hypnosis	Hypotension Respiratory depression Paradoxical agitation Hyprosmolar metabolic acidosis due to drug solvent at escalating or high doses	Increase doses slowly by increments with titration. Monitor blood pressure and respiratory status. Administer fluids as indicated. With escalating or high-dose therapy, monitor daily and total doses for drug and propylene glycol solvent. Slowly wean from drug after prologed therapy.
Nonbenzodiazepine sedative			
Propofol	Anxiolysis, amnesia, hypnosis	Hypotension Hyperlipidemia Respiratory depression Infection risk from lapses in aseptic technique	Patient must be intubated and receiving mechanical ventilation. Monitor blood pressure and hemodynamic status. Use aseptic technique when handling drug. Change infusion set every 12 hours. Monitor plasma lipid levels. Increase or decrease infusion incrementally to specific sedation level. Avoid abrupt discontinuation of drug.
Neuroleptic			
Haloperidol	Antipsychotic effects, antidelirium effects	Extrapyramidal effects Neuroleptic malignant syndrome Prolonged QT interval Torsades de pointes	Measure QT interval at start of therapy and periodically. Use with caution when patient is receiving other proarrhythmic agents. Administer anticholinergic as indicated if extrapyramidal effects occur.
Narcotics			
Morphine	Analgesia, relief of air hunger	Hypotension Gastrointestinal hypomotility Respiratory depression Nausea and vomiting Histamine release Itching or rash Urinary retention	Increase doses slowly by increments with titration. Monitor blood pressure and respiratory status. Administer fluids as indicated. Slowly wean from drug after prolonged therapy.
Fentanyl	Analgesia, relief of air hunger	Hypotension Gastrointestinal hypomotility Respiratory depression Muscle rigidity Bradycardia Itching	Increase doses slowly by increments with titration. Monitor blood pressure, heart rate, and respiratory status. Administer fluids as indicated. Give as an infusion if extended therapy is required. Slowly wean from drug after prolonged therapy.
Dilaudid	Analgesia, relief of air hunger	Hypotension Gastrointestinal hypomotility Respiratory depression	Increase doses slowly by increments with titration. Monitor blood pressure and respiratory status. Administer fluids as indicated.
Meperidine	Analygesia, relief of air hunger	Hypotension Gastrointestinal hypomotility Respiratory depression Tachycardia Seizures Urinary retention	Increase doses slowly by increments with titration. Monitor blood pressure and respiratory status. Administer fluids as indicated. Avoid using in the intensive care unit, particularly high doses or prolonged use.
Remifentanil	Analygesia	Hypotension Gastrointestinal hypomotility Respiratory depression Muscle rigidity Bradycardia Itching	Increase doses slowly by increments with titration. Monitor blood pressure and respiratory status. Administer fluids as indicated. Give as a infusion because of the short duration of action.

Reprinted with permission.[6p53]

setting, upward titration of opioid analgesia is absolutely appropriate even though side effects of opioid analgesics such as sedation and cardiopulmonary depression may occur and hasten death. The key point is that opioid analgesia is used for the primary purpose of relieving pain and suffering. Without such intervention, pain such as that experienced during the terminal phase of some types of cancer is frequently undertreated.[31] There is a moral, ethical, and legal responsibility on the part of health care professionals to aggressively treat pain, even if dose requirements to relieve distress and suffering are much higher than those needed only for pain relief. In addition, patients previously treated with opioid analgesics usually have developed a tolerance to this drug class, requiring much higher opioid dosing to achieve the same clinical effect.[32]

History of Substance Abuse

Patients with substance abuse issues present challenges in providing optimal analgesia in the critical care unit. One challenge is that tolerance to opioids may have developed following long-term exposure to that drug class. Ultimately this may require far higher than standard opioid dosing. Often health care providers may be reluctant to prescribe or administer nonstandard opioid doses. A second challenge is that of stereotyping a patient. Patients with a known history of substance abuse may be perceived as drug seeking, leading health care providers to be reluctant to adequately treat expressed pain. The patient's report of pain remains the gold standard for pain assessment. As such, analgesic administration and titration should be based on what the patient says is his or her pain as well as effectiveness of interventions, especially if the patient is acutely ill or injured.

It is also important to differentiate between tolerance, physical dependence, addiction/abuse, and pseudo-addiction and drug withdrawal. *Tolerance* represents a physiologic response to a given drug dosing where upward drug titration is required to maintain the same clinical effect. *Physical dependence* refers to the onset of withdrawal symptoms following abrupt interruption of opioid analgesia. This typically is associated with tolerance. *Addiction/abuse* refers to a psychologic and behavioral syndrome characterized by drug craving and compulsive use despite physical, psychologic, or social harm to the user. *Pseudo-addiction* refers to behaviors that clinicians may associate with addiction, such as requests for higher opioid doses, but which is actually caused by inadequate pain management.[14,33]

Pain in the Elderly Patient

People older than 65 years of age are expected to be greater than 20% of the population in 2050. This demographic change is reflected in the aging of the population in acute and critical care settings.[34,35] Management of critical illness in the elderly is complicated by multiple factors, including reduced physiologic reserve, nutritional issues, and a host of age-related changes in end-organ function affecting responses to drug therapy. Drug absorption, distribution, metabolism, and elimination are typically altered in the elderly patient.[36] Thus the elderly are at risk for more prolonged and profound clinical effects from a given drug dosing. To minimize these consequences, opioid analgesics should be administered in small increments and utilized to achieve appropriate analgesia with the lowest dose possible.[6]

Discussion of opioid therapy must also include mention of cognitive side effects. Cognitive function refers to the brain's ability to acquire, process, store, and retrieve information. Following opioid administration many patients report a subjective sense of mental dullness. Changes in cognitive function are not limited to self-reports of "mental dullness" but may include development of hypoactive or hyperactive delirium as a side effect of therapy.[37] For these reasons, patient assessment following opioid administration cannot be limited to determinations of adequacy of analgesia but must also include ongoing assessment of mental status due to risks associated with delirium. The elderly population is typically at higher risk for this complication of therapy as an adverse drug reaction.

Research Applications

Much of the more recent research into pain has been undertaken in acute care settings or involving pain interventions. Some of this research can be applied to critical care practice, but this must be done cautiously.

Pain Assessment in the Cognitively Impaired

Recognizing that pain is a subjective experience, affected by multiple factors, further attention is being paid to nonverbal indications of pain seen in an increasing variety of patient populations, including patients with cancer,[38,39] elderly patients with dementia, and those who are ventilated and sedated.[40] The gold standard for pain assessment, the patient's self-report, is clearly compromised in the cognitively impaired patient. Therefore, research has involved evaluation and validation of pain behaviors to make decisions regarding analgesic therapy in the cognitively impaired.

In the American Association of Critical-Care Nurses (AACN) Thunder Project 2, specific pain-related behaviors associated with painful procedures were correlated with patient verbal self-report of pain. Establishing validity and reliability of nonverbal cues to pain through scientific inquiry is very significant in terms of pain assessment and intervention in patients who are cognitively impaired, sedated, or receiving controlled ventilation.[5] Meta-analytic techniques across multiple studies involving assessment of acute pain have established a temporal relationship and correlation between acute pain, verbal self-reports of pain intensity, and pain behaviors.[41]

Pain at End of Life

Pain management in palliative care situations is receiving increasing attention and is one of the pain goals in the End-of-Life Nursing Education Consortium.[42] Assessing pain at the end of life may be complicated by equivocal physical assessment findings, lethargy, disease progression, and tolerance to drug therapy. With honest, open communication among the team members, family, and patient, terminal sedation may be appropriate for relief of suffering.[43]

Gender and Pain Management

Pain may be mediated by gender role socialization, cognitive and affective factors in pain behaviors, as well as pain self-reporting.[44] Baseline anxiety and gender are also reported to modulate the pain response. In one study, higher anxiety may predict more pain relief among males versus females due to sex differences in individualized coping strategies or placebo effects.[45] Biochemical and neurohumoral responses to painful stress also change based on sex. A larger increase in serum cortisol levels are noted in men following painful stimulation.[46]

Gastrointestinal (GI) Hypomotility Related to Opioid Analgesia

Methylnaltrexone is a long-acting opioid antagonist that does not cross the blood-brain barrier. Administered IV or via the GI tract, it had been shown to be effective in reversing opioid-induced GI dysfunction while not producing systemic opioid withdrawal.[47-49] Naloxone, administered via the GI tract, has also been effective in reversing opioid-induced GI dysfunction while not producing precipitous opioid withdrawal symptoms.[50] Most of the populations studied to date have been utilizing long-acting agents outside of the critical care setting; however, the physiology behind opioid-induced GI hypomotility is the same between populations.

In a critically ill patient, opioid-induced GI hypomotility may be treated by a number of techniques including aggressive bowel regimens, close monitoring and management of fluid intake through the GI tract, and observation of tolerance to feeds. In addition, medications to promote GI motility such as metocloropromide may be considered. In patients refractory to these techniques, it may be appropriate to consider using a selective opioid antagonist or administration technique. These are designed to avoid significant opioid antagonism in the CNS (and maintain analgesia) while antagonizing opioid occupancy of peripheral receptors such as those in the gut, thus treating opioid-induced GI hypomotility. If this treatment option is utilized, patients must be monitored closely for therapeutic effect (laxation response) as well as side effects.

More recently, studies in the adult population have examined alternative routes of administration for opioid therapy[51] as well as the influence of age on drug pharmacokinetics and pharmacodynamics.[52] The question of whether and to what degree the elderly patient is receiving best practice in assessment and management of pain is paramount in this vulnerable population.[53] Pain management using interven-

tional procedures such as site-specific delivery of local anesthetic agents, central neuroaxis administration of therapy, and regional techniques are being increasingly studied in acutely and critically ill adults.[3,8,54-58] Pain management using topical applications of pharmacologic agents is being studied in neuropathic pain states.[59] Research also suggests that education, both for clinicians as well as patients, is still necessary due to fears of addiction among surgical patients.[60]

Barriers to Pain Management

A number of barriers exist to adequate pain management in general.[5,14,16,38,40-41,53,60] These include:

- Consumer belief that pain is to be expected and endured ("no pain, no gain"), a general reluctance to report pain, and fears that use of opioid analgesics will lead to addiction ("just say no")
- Compromised or equivocal physical assessment in the nonverbal patient
- Reluctance to aggressively treat pain in terminal or palliative care situations for fear of shortening the patient's life
- Individual health care providers' lack of knowledge of pain management or biases related to pain management in selected populations such as those addicted to opioids
- Barriers to pain management also exist regarding assessing the specific type of pain being experienced by the patient. Neuropathic pain has a different physiologic basis than nociceptive pain and is more effectively treated by sodium channel blockers or adjunctive agents rather than by systemic opioids as is the case with nociceptive pain.
- Health care and governmental systems also create barriers to adequate pain management due to:
  - Failure to include outcomes related to pain management in quality review programs
  - Legislation and institutional policies that require additional paperwork to provide certain analgesic medications and therapies
  - Disputes on distribution of reimbursement for pain management services
  - Restrictions on options for pain management

Health care practitioners must be aware of these barriers, and must work with patients and within the community to eliminate the deleterious effects of the barriers on patients' care and outcomes.

In critical care, many critical care practitioners are unaware of patients' discomfort or are unaware of the physiologic effects of pain. Attention may be focused on other potentially life-threatening problems, and pain assessments may be done less frequently. Many critically ill patients cannot communicate their pain verbally because they are intubated, chemically paralyzed, or sedated. Without a verbal complaint of pain, there is risk of critical care practitioners not recognizing the presence of pain and missing the relationship between pain, physiologic stress, and nonverbal pain behaviors.[1,5,15]

A barrier also exists to optimal pain management with regard to adequate dosing of analgesics. A patient being treated in a critical care setting who has a preexisting tolerance to opioid analgesics may legitimately require higher-than-standard doses to achieve optimal analgesia. The concept of "dosing to effect" comes into play here and justifies high-dose therapy as indicated. Lastly, many practitioners may not recognize that anxiety may increase pain perception, and pain increases anxiety. In this setting, it may be appropriate, with close monitoring and careful patient selection, to dose with multiple drug classes such as a benzodiazepine and opioid agents. The synergistic effect from careful titration of both drug classes may have a dramatic dose-sparing effect, potentially protecting the patient from side effects of both forms of therapy.

APPLICATION OF SCIENTIFIC KNOWLEDGE TO PRACTICE

The following questions should repeatedly be asked and answered in order to provide adequate pain management in critical care.

Who is at risk for pain? Although any critically ill patient may be expected to experience pain, the following patients are at particular risk: patients who have medical conditions that include ischemic, infectious, or inflammatory processes; are immobilized; have wounds; have invasive therapeutic or monitoring devices in place; are undergoing procedures of any type; or those who have sustained traumatic injury. Nurses should plan preemptive use of analgesia in all these situations in which pain is likely. A patient with a history of diabetes and potential metabolic injury is at risk for neuropathic pain and should be assessed and treated accordingly.

Who is at risk for poor pain management? Nurses should be aware of patients' characteristics that may interfere with the ability to communicate pain. Health care professionals should avoid biases that may cause them to miss clues or undertreat obvious pain (Table 6-3).

Who is the best source of information about the pain experienced? The answer is the patient. If a patient cannot verbally tell someone about the pain, body language and physiologic status can provide clues to the presence of pain (Table 6-4). However, nonverbal behaviors should never be used instead of, or to refute, a patient's verbal complaint of pain. Patient history should also be reviewed for potential chronic pain issues as well as concurrent drug therapy that may contribute to tolerance to analgesics.

How should pain be assessed? To be clinically useful, a pain assessment method must be reliable and valid, easy for patients to use, and easy for providers to administer and interpret. Numerical rating scales, visual analogue scales, and descriptive rating scales meet these requirements and

---

Table 6-3   Factors Associated with Undertreatment of Pain in Critically Ill and Injured Patients

- Focus of health care providers on life-threatening problems
- Infrequent assessment of pain
- Health care providers' lack of awareness of the physiological effects of pain
- Desensitization of health care providers to pain inflicted by needed procedures
- Patients' inability to communicate because of intubation, sedation, and chemical paralysis
- Patients' assumption that pain must be endured, that everything that can be done is being done
- Inadequate focus on relationship between pain and anxiety
- Inadequate awareness of weight-based dosing
- Patient history and physical assessment not sufficiently thorough, which may potentially result in standard opioid dosing inadequate for patient needs due to preexisting substance abuse or medication history with resulting high tolerance for opioid analgesics.
- Inadequate awareness of cardiopulmonary instability with resulting reluctance to dose adequately to treat pain.
- Poor understanding of neuropathic pain, inadequate treatment
- Inadequate awareness of nonverbal pain behaviors
- Inadequate recognition of activities, procedures, and stimuli that may be perceived as painful by the patient
- Dementia
- Language barrier

Table 6-4   Behavioral Cues to Acute Pain

Type of Behavior	Examples
Facial expression	Grimacing, clenching teeth, tightly shutting lips, gazing/staring, wrinkling forehead, tearing, wincing, shutting of eyes
Vocalization	Moaning, groaning, grunting, sighing, gasping, crying, screaming
Verbalization	Praying, counting, swearing/cursing, repeating nonsensical phrases
Body action	Thrashing, pounding, biting, rocking, rubbing, clenching of fists
Coping behaviors	Massaging, immobilizing, guarding, bracing, eating/drinking, applying pressure/heat/cold, assuming a special position or posture, reading, watching television, listening to music

Reprinted by permission from Puntillo K, Wilkie D. Assessment of pain in the critically ill. In: Puntillo K, ed. *Pain in the Critically Ill: Assessment and Management.* Gaithersburg, Md: Aspen; 1991:54.

---

are available in a variety of forms for use with adults (see Appendixes 6A and 6B).

When should pain be assessed? Pain should be assessed on a regular schedule around the clock. For example, in a critical care setting, every 2 hours or more frequently, and following any interventions so that effectiveness may be assessed. Pain should be assessed before and after procedures. It should also be assessed at an appropriate time after a therapeutic intervention, for example, at the time when the patient might be expected to sense the onset or peak effects of an analgesic medication. This assessment should also be agent specific. For example, the peak effects of fentanyl citrate occur within as little as 2-3 minutes, and the peak effect of morphine sulfate may not occur for 10 minutes or longer.

When should analgesic therapy be started? Ideally, analgesic therapy should be started before pain begins (preemptive analgesia) or as soon as possible after pain is recognized. For acute pain, analgesic therapies should initially be provided on a regular schedule around the clock or possibly by continuous infusion with close titration. To prevent the onset of pain, the patient may need to be awakened to receive a regularly scheduled dose of analgesic or a treatment. Drugs with a relatively short duration of action, for example 3 to 6 hours, are used so that doses can be titrated to effect. Additional doses or treatments should be available as needed for episodes of increased pain. As the acute pain decreases, analgesic therapies can be changed to an as-needed basis. For chronic pain and pain associated with cancer, analgesic treatments should cover the entire 24-hour period. This around-the-clock approach should include use of long-acting medications supplemented by as-needed doses or treatments for breakthrough pain.

What methods should be used? Type of pain, severity of pain, and patients' preferences should be considered in selecting methods of pain management. In general, pharmacologic and nonpharmacologic methods should be used together to manage pain. Analgesic methods that interrupt impulse transmission peripherally (eg, heat or cold, NSAIDs) should be used in combination with centrally acting therapies (eg, relaxation, opioids). Adjunctive therapies may be more appropriate to use with neuropathic pain.

The World Health Organization recommends the use of a stepped approach to the use of analgesics (see Figure 6-1). For mild pain, acetaminophen or NSAIDs should be the first therapy. For moderate to severe pain, opioid analgesics are the initial therapy, preferably administered intravenously (see Appendix 6C).

Patients should be carefully screened for characteristics that would preclude the use of selected analgesic medications. For example, patients with impaired renal function and patients more than 65 years old should have doses of NSAIDs reduced or withheld. Patients who are hypovolemic should not receive continuous infusions of opioids until adequate fluid volume can be established. Once initial pain control is gained, additional analgesic technologies such as epidural infusion or patient-controlled analgesia (PCA) can be added to maintain the patient's comfort. For long-term opioid therapy, with good patient selection, transdermal delivery systems such as fentanyl transdermal systems may provide a stable, long-term plasma concentration of the drug and a stable analgesic state.

In addition, nonpharmacologic methods (Table 6-5)

Figure 6-1 Three-step analgesic ladder. Reproduced by permission of WHO from *Cancer Pain Relief,* 2nd ed. Geneva: WHO; 1996.

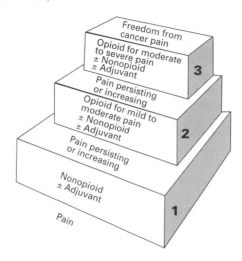

should be incorporated into the treatment plan as tolerated by the patient. Physical methods work in 1 of 2 ways. They may minimize further pathophysiologic processes such as inflammation or decrease active stimulation of nociceptors in the injured area, or they stimulate other benign peripheral nerve impulses that block the transmission of nociceptive impulses in the dorsal horn of the spinal cord. Cognitive and behavioral methods may enable patients to harness the power of the mind and change thoughts, emotions, and physiologic responses to pain. Successful use of cognitive

Table 6-5	**Nonpharmacologic Analgesic Therapies**
Physical Therapies	
Application of heat or cold	
Positioning or elevation	
External support or immobilization	
Cutaneous vibration or transcutaneous electrical nerve stimulation	
Massage	
Acupressure or acupuncture	
Slow, controlled repositioning	
Avoidance of contact with pressure points/bony prominences	
Healing touch	
Aromatherapy	
Cognitive and Behavioral Therapies	
Distraction (auditory, visual, tactile, rhythmic)	
Relaxation or biofeedback	
Guided imagery	
Hypnosis or meditation	
Patient teaching or preparatory information	
Yoga	
Active listening	

and behavioral methods requires various levels of attention, discipline, training, and practice and a controlled environment. For these reasons, these methods are not generally practical in a critical care setting. However some methods, such as distraction and simple relaxation, may be immediately applicable in acute situations. Brief instructional scripts can be used to assist patients with these techniques (see Appendix 6D).

To maximize success in healing pain management, health care professionals should do the following:

1. Assess the patient. Each person is unique. Assess for pain severity, location, intensity, quality, and type.
2. Plan pain management to prevent pain.
3. Involve the patient when possible, and communicate expectations of therapy realistically. Educate patients about the goals of therapy.
4. Combine pharmacologic and nonpharmacologic therapies based on peripheral and central mechanisms of action.
5. Use a flowsheet to document responses to therapy and the adjustments made.
6. Never give up in seeking solutions to resolve pain. Seek out persons within the institution (eg, advanced practice nurse, pharmacologist, anesthesiologist, pain management team) who can help.

COMPETENCY

Every licensed nurse should demonstrate competency in assessing and managing acute pain. Nurses who practice in specialty areas such as burn, rehabilitation, neurology, and oncology units should become competent in assessing and managing more difficult pain syndromes. These competencies can be developed through a variety of means. Background knowledge can be gained in undergraduate education, by reading journal articles, and by participating in formal and informal classes. Clinical skills can be developed by guided clinical practice with more experienced nurses and with members of institutional pain management teams.

ETHICAL CONSIDERATIONS

Even patients chemically paralyzed or deeply sedated may be at risk for awareness, conscious perception of pain, and physiologic consequences of pain. Patients may be able to sense and interpret hearing, touch, and movement. These findings indicate the importance of providing analgesic therapies to even apparently unaware or unresponsive patients.

Analgesic therapies must also be provided to patients with histories of substance abuse. Pain may be difficult to control in these patients and require higher-than-standard opioid dosing, but failure to provide appropriate, adequate pain control is unethical. Lack of pain relief also places additional physiologic and psychologic burdens on the patient at a time when these functions are already stressed.

FUTURE RESEARCH

Additional research in critical care settings is needed. Studies should be done to determine if, and in what ways, pain and pain management in critically ill and injured patients differs from pain and pain management in less acutely ill and injured patients. Results of these studies could be used to determine the practicality and extent to which results from research in acutely ill patients can be extrapolated to the care of critically ill patients.

Priority should also be assigned to studies that focus on the following areas related to pain in critically ill patients:

- Pain assessment, particularly in patients unable to give a verbal report
- The prevalence, extent, and relief of pain associated with commonly performed procedures
- The safety and effectiveness of pharmacologic and nonpharmacologic therapies
- Incidence and prevalence of neuropathic pain in acute and critical care settings that requires a different pharmacologic approach for effective treatment

REFERENCES

1. Hamill-Ruth RJ, Marohn ML. Evaluation of pain in the critically ill patient. *Crit Care Clin.* 1999;15(1):35-54.
2. Mularski RA. Pain management in the intensive care unit. *Crit Care Clin.* 2004;20:381-401.
3. Heavner JE, Willis WD. Pain pathways: anatomy and physiology. In: Raj PP, ed. *Practical Management of Pain.* 3rd ed. St. Louis, Mo; Mosby Inc; 2000.
4. Johnson BW. Pain mechanisms: anatomy, physiology, and neurochemistry. In: Raj PP, ed. *Practical Management of Pain.* 3rd ed. St. Louis, Mo; Mosby Inc; 2000.
5. Puntillo KA, Morris AB, Thompson CL, Stanik-Hutt J, White CA, Wild LR. Pain behaviors observed during six common procedures: results from Thunder Project II. *Crit Care Med.* 2004;32(2):421-427.
6. Arbour RB. Sedation and pain management in critically ill adults. *Crit Care Nurse.* 2000;20(5):39-56.
7. Woolf CJ, Max MB. Mechanism-based pain diagnosis. *Anesthiology.* 2001;95(1):241-249.
8. Matot I, Drenger B, Weissman C, Shauli A, Gozal Y. Epidural clonidine, bupivicaine and methadone as the sole analgesic agent after thoracotomy for lung resection. *Anaesthesia.* 2004;59:861-866.
9. Epstein J, Breslow MJ. The stress response of critical illness. *Crit Care Clin.* 1999;15(1):17-33.
10. Lang JD. Pain: a prelude. *Crit Care Clin.* 1999;15(1):1-16.
11. McArdle P. Intravenous analgesia. *Crit Care Clin.* 1999;15(1);89-104.
12. Piacentine L, Maloni H, Mogensen K, et al. Pain and headaches. In: Bader MK, Littlejohns LR, eds. *AANN*

Core Curriculum for Neuroscience Nursing. St. Louis, Mo: Elsevier Inc; 2004.

13. Merskey M, Bogduk N. *International Association for the Study of Pain: Task Force on Taxonomy, Classification of Chronic Pain.* 2nd ed. Seattle, Wash: IASP Press; 1994.

14. McCaffery M, Pasero C. Assessment: Underlying complexities, misconceptions and practical tools. In: McCaffrey M, Pasero C, eds. *Pain: Clinical Manual.* 2nd ed. St Louis, Mo. Mosby Inc; 1999:35-102.

15. Odhner M, Wegman D, Freeland N, Steinmetz, L, Ingersoll G. Assessing pain control in nonverbal critically ill adults. *Dimens Crit Care Nurs.* 2003;22:260-267.

16. Puntillo K. Pain assessment and management in the critically ill: wizardry or science? *Am J Crit Care.* 2003; 12(4):310-316.

17. Arbour R. Using bispectral index monitoring to detect potential breakthrough awareness and limit duration of neuromuscular blockade. *Am J Crit Care.* 2004;13(1): 66-73.

18. Gallagher RM. The pain-depression conundrum: bridging the body and mind. Available at: http://www.medscape.com/viewprogram/2030. Accessed September 10, 2002.

19. Manning DC. Outcomes, efficacy and complications of neuropathic pain therapy. In: Raj PP, ed. *Practical Management of Pain.* 3rd ed. St. Louis, Mo; Mosby Inc; 2000.

20. Katz JA. Nonsteroidal anti-inflammatory agents. In: Raj PP, ed. *Practical Management of Pain.* 3rd ed. St. Louis, Mo; Mosby Inc; 2000.

21. Medscape Drug Information. Ketorolac tromethamine injection: pharmacology and chemistry. Available at: http://www.medscape.com/druginfo/search?searchfor=Clinical&cid=med&search_type=drug&queryText=ketorolac%20tromethamine%20injection:%20pharmacology%20chemistry. Accessed June 12, 2003.

22. Mycek MJ, Harvey RA, Champe PC. *Lippincott's Illustrated Reviews: Pharmacology.* 2nd ed. Philadelphia, Pa: J B Lippincott; 1997:133-142,401-418.

23. Hedderich R, Ness TJ. Analgesia for trauma and burns. *Crit Care Clin.* 1999;15(1):167-184.

24. Murray MJ, DeRuyter ML, Harrison BA. Opioids and benzodiazepines. *Crit Care Clin.* 1995;11(4):849-872.

25. Mandabach MG. Intrathecal and epidural analgesia. *Crit Care Clin.* 1999;15(1):105-118.

26. Staats PS, Dougherty PM. Spinal analgesics: present and future. In: Raj PP, ed. *Practical Management of Pain.* 3rd ed. St. Louis, Mo; Mosby Inc; 2000.

27. Burton AW, Eappen S. Regional anesthesia techniques for pain control in the intensive care unit. *Crit Care Clin.* 1999;15(1):77-89.

28. Levetown M. Palliative care in the intensive care unit. *New Horiz.* 1998;6(4):383-397.

29. Kvale PA, Simoff MS, Prakash UBS. Palliative care. *Chest.* 2003;123(1):284S-311S.

30. Schwarz JK. The rule of double effect and its role in facilitating good end-of-life palliative care. *J Hosp Pall Nurs.* 2004;6(2):125-133.

31. Dahl JL. Effective pain management in terminal care. *Clin in Geriat Med.* 1996;12(2):279-300.

32. Civetta JM. Critical palliative care: intensive care redefined. *Surg Oncol Clin North Am.* 2001;10(1):137-159.

33. Swica Y, Breitbart W. Treating pain in patients with AIDS and a history of substance use. *West J Med.* 2002; 176(1):33-39.

34. Lynch D. Geriatric pain. In: Raj PP, ed. *Practical Management of Pain.* 3rd ed. St. Louis, Mo; Mosby Inc; 2000.

35. Tolley G, Prevost S. Case management of critically ill elders: a case study. *AACN Clin Issues.* 1997;8(4):635-642.

36. Neilson C. Pharmacologic considerations in critical care of the elderly. *Clin Geri Med.* 1994;10(1):71-89.

37. Ersek M, Cherrier MM, Overman SS, Irving GA. The cognitive effects of opioids. *Pain Manag Nurs.* 2004; 5(2):75-93.

38. Soscia J. Assessing pain in cognitively impaired older adults with cancer. *Clin J Oncol Nurs.* 2003;7(2):174-177.

39. Turk DC, Monarch ES, Williams AD. Cancer patients in pain: considerations for assessing the whole person. *Hemat Oncol Clin North Am.* 2002;16(3):511-525.

40. Manfredi PL, Breuer B, Meier DE, Libow L. Pain assessment in elderly patients with severe dementia. *J Pain Symptom Manage.* 2003;25(1):48-52.

41. Labus JS, Keefe FJ, Jensen MP. Self-reports of pain intensity and direct observations of pain behavior: when are they correlated? *Pain.* 2003;102(1-2):109-124.

42. Sherman DW, Matzo ML, Paice JA, McLaughlin M, Virani R. Learning pain assessment and management: a goal of the End-of-Life Nursing Education Consortium. *J Contin Educ Nurs.* 2004;35(3):107-119.

43. Panke JT. Difficulties in managing pain at the end of life. *Am J Nurs.* 2002;102(7):26-34.

44. Myers CD, Riley JL, Robinson ME. Psychosocial contributions to sex related differences in pain. *Clin J Pain.* 2003;19(4):225-232.

45. Edwards R, Augustson E, Fillingim R. Differential relationships between anxiety and treatment-associated pain reduction among male and female chronic pain patients. *Clin J Pain.* 2003;19(4):208-216.

46. Zimmer C, Basler HD, Vedder H, Lautenbacher S. Sex differences in cortisol responses to noxious stress. *Clin J Pain.* 2003;19(4):233-239.

47. Foss JF. A review of the potential role of methylnaltrexone in opioid bowel dysfunction. *Am J Surg.* 2001;182 (5A suppl):19S-26S.

48. Friedman JD, Dello Buono FA. Opioid antagonists in the treatment of opioid-induced constipation and pruritus. *Ann Pharmacother.* 2001;35(1):85-91.

49. Yuan CS, Foss JF, O'Connor M, et al. Methylnaltrex-

one for reversal of constipation due to chronic methadone use: a randomized controlled trial. *JAMA.* 2000;282(3): 367-372.

50. Meissner W, Schmidt U, Hartmann M, et al. Oral naloxone reverses opioid-associated constipation. *Pain.* 2000; 84(1):105-109.

51. Zeppetella G. An assessment of the safety, efficacy and acceptability of intranasal fentanyl citrate in the management of cancer-related breakthrough pain: a pilot study. *J Pain Symptom Manag.* 2000;20(4):253-258.

52. Kharasch ED, Hoffer C, Whittington D. Influence of age on the pharmacokinetics and pharmacodynamics of oral transmucosal fentanyl citrate. *Anesthesiology.* 2004;101(3):738-743.

53. Herr K, Titler MG, Schilling ML, et al. Evidence-based assessment of acute pain in older adults: current nursing practices and perceived barriers. *Clin J Pain.* 2004;20(5): 331-340.

54. Deer T, Chappel I, Classen A, et al. Intrathecal drug delivery for treatment of chronic low back pain: report from the national outcomes registry for low back pain. *Pain Med.* 2004;5(1):6-13.

55. Ilfeld BM, Thannikary LJ, Morey TE, Vander Griend RA, Ennekind FK. Popliteal sciatic perineural local anesthetic infusion. *Anesthesiology.* 2004;101(4):970-977.

56. Manabe H, Dan K, Hirata K, et al. Optimum pain relief with continuous epidural infusion of local anesthetics shortens the duration of zoster-associated pain. *Clin J Pain.* 2004;20(5):302-308.

57. Moraca RJ, Sheldon DG, Thirlby RC. The role of epidural anesthesia and analgesia in surgical practice. *Ann Surg.* 2003;238(5):663-673.

58. Yamamuro M, Kusaka K, Kato M, Takahashi M. Celiac plexus block in cancer pain management. *Tohoku J Exper Med.* 2000;192(1):1-18.

59. Lynch ME, Clark AJ, Sawynok J. A pilot study examining topical amitryptyline, ketamine and a combination of both in the treatment of neuropathic pain. *Clin J Pain.* 2003;19(5):323-328.

60. Greer SM, Dalton J, Carlson J, Youngblood R. Surgical patients' fear of addiction to pain medication: the effect of an educational program for clinicians. *Clin J Pain.* 2001;17(2):157-164.

SUGGESTED READINGS

1. American Pain Society. *Principles of Analgesic Use in the Treatment of Acute Pain and Cancer Pain.* 5th ed. Skokie, Ill: American Pain Society; 2003.

2. American Society of Pain Management Nurses; St. Marie B, ed. *Core Curriculum for Pain Management Nursing.* St. Louis, Mo: W B Saunders Co; 2002.

3. De Jonghe B, Bastuji-Garin S, Fangio P. et al. Sedation algorithm in critically ill patients without acute brain injury. *Crit Care Med.* 2005;33(1):120-127.

4. Hanks-Bell M, Halvey K, Paice JA. Pain assessment and management in aging. *Online J Issues Nurs.* Available at: http://www.medscape.com/viewarticle/490773. Accessed December 20, 2004.

5. Keller S, Bann CM, Dodd SL, Schein J, Mendoza TR, Cleeland CS. Validity of the brief pain inventory for use in documenting the outcomes of patients with non-cancer pain. *Clin J Pain.* 2004;20(5):309-318.

6. Kollef MH, Levy NT, Ahrens TS, Schiaff RS, Prentice D, Sherman G. The use of continuous IV sedation is associated with prolongation of mechanical ventilation. *Chest.* 1998;114:541-548.

7. Kress JP, Pohlman AS, O'Connor MF, Hall JB. Daily interruption of sedative infusions in critically ill patients undergoing mechanical ventilation. *New Engl J Med.* 2000;342(20):1471-1477.

8. McCaffrey M. Pain control: switching from IV to PO. *Am J Nurs.* 2003;103(5):62-64.

9. Mascia MF, Koch M, Medicis JJ. Pharmacoeconomic impact of rational use guidelines on the provision of analgesia, sedation and neuromuscular blockade in critical care. *Crit Care Med.* 2000;28(7):2300-2306.

10. Moraca RJ, Sheldon DG, Thirlby RC. The role of epidural anesthesia and analgesia in surgical practice. *Ann Surg.* 2003;238(5):663-673.

11. National Pharmaceutical Council, Inc, Joint Commission of Accreditation of Healthcare Organizations. Pain: current understanding of assessment, management and treatments. Available at: http://www.npcnow.org/resources/PDFs/PainAddendum.pdf. Accessed December 27, 2004.

12. Raj PP, ed. *Practical Management of Pain.* 3rd ed. St. Louis, Mo; Mosby Inc 2000.

13. Webster LR. Assessing abuse potential in pain patients. Medscape Neurology and Neurosurgery. Available at: http://www.medscape.com/viewarticle/471663. Accessed April 7, 2004.

CLINICAL RECOMMENDATIONS

The rating scale for the Level of Recommendation ranges from I to VI, with levels indicated as follows: I, manufacturer's recommendations only; II, theory based, no research data to support recommendations; recommendations from expert consensus group may exist; III, laboratory data only, no clinical data to support recommendations; IV, limited clinical studies to support recommendations; V, clinical studies in more than 1 or 2 different populations and situations to support recommendations; VI, clinical studies in a variety of patient populations and situations to support recommendations.

Pain Management in the Acutely and Critically Ill

Period of Use	Recommendations	Rationale for Recommendation	Level of Recommendation	Supporting References	Comments
Selection of Patients at Risk for Pain	Consider *all* patients in the acute and critical care environment at risk for pain due to illness, procedures, positioning, airway manipulation, controlled ventilation and suctioning, or metabolic injury to peripheral nervous system.	Patients are at risk for pain when unconscious, sedated, mechanically ventilated, or chemically paralyzed. Anxiety is a common consequence of critical illness, which increases pain perception. Even routine nursing care activities are known to cause pain. Patients may not appear to be in pain when in fact they are.	VI: Clinical studies in a variety of populations and situations	See Annotated Bibliography: 3, 4, 7, 10 See Other References: 1, 2, 3, 5, 6, 9, 15, 18, 23, 25, 31, 45, 54, 57, 59, 62, 63 See References: 1, 2, 4, 23, 33, 39 See Suggested Readings: 1, 2, 11, 12	Common devices and procedures used in the critical care environment and reported as painful by patients include the following: • Chest, nasogastric, and endotracheal tube insertion and removal; pneumatic compression devices; arterial and central venous catheters; and external skeletal fixators as well as peripheral venipuncture and wound care/dressing changes and invasive drain removal • Turning, coughing, deep breathing, walking, and range-of-motion exercises
Assessment	Acknowledge that the patient is the best judge of his or her pain. Verbal self-report of pain remains the gold standard but pain assessment can be *significantly* augmented by assessing nonverbal pain behaviors or vocalization in patients who are not cognitively intact such as sedated patients, those with dementia, or those with CNS injury.	The verbal self-report is the gold standard for pain assessment. Pain entails a subjective and physiologic response to noxious stimuli. Response is affected by age, cultural background, past experience, and type of stimuli. Response is also affected by ability of the patient to interact, type of injury, and concurrent drug therapy. In addition, sleep deprivation with resultant increase in anxiety may increase pain perception.	VI: Clinical studies in a variety of populations and situations	See Annotated Bibliography: 1, 5, 6, 7 See Other References: 1, 3, 20, 44, 45, 50, 66 See References: 1, 2, 5, 6, 14-17, 34-36, 38, 40-43, 53 See Suggested Readings: 2, 4, 11	Endorphin levels in patients can vary a great deal. Endorphins are the body's internal opioids. This variation is one explanation of the great variety of responses to the same intensity of noxious stimuli in different patients. Pain assessment may be difficult in a nonverbal patient. Identification of pain location or intensity may need to be based on nonverbal behaviors such as grimacing or motor tension.

Period of Use	Recommendations	Rationale for Recommendation	Level of Recommendation	Supporting References	Comments
Assessment (*cont.*)	With good patient selection and family interaction, a close family member may possibly serve as a surrogate for the patient when determining pain response behaviors. This may be appropriate in circumstances where the patient is nonverbal and long-term family caregivers are familiar with the patients' nonverbal pain behaviors. Evaluate and document the following parameters of pain: • Location • Intensity • Qualitative characteristics • Aggravating and alleviating factors • Associated signs and symptoms, pain behaviors. • Patterns of pain related to incidence, intensity	Assessment of each parameter is necessary to obtain the best pain diagnosis. A patient may be hospitalized for a specific purpose, such as a surgical procedure, but may have pain related to other chronic conditions (eg, arthritis), complications, or additional acute conditions such as intraoperative myocardial infarction. Pain may also result from metabolic injury to peripheral nerves or complications of therapy such as neuropathic pain following cancer chemotherapy.	V: Clinical studies in more than 1 or 2 different patient populations to support recommendations.	See Other References: 3, 9, 13, 15, 44, 45, 47, 48, 53, 62 See References: 1, 2, 5, 6, 14-17, 34-36, 38, 40-43, 53 See Suggested Readings: 2, 4, 11	Qualitative characteristics include the patient's description of his or her pain, nonverbal behaviors, and the ascribed meaning of the pain to the patient. Associated signs and symptoms include physiologic changes in vital signs, nausea, and vomiting. Vital sign changes as pain indicators *must* be interpreted with caution as they can be affected by clinical state, fluid status, and concurrent drug therapy. Also, vital signs may be at the patients' baseline, and the patient may still be experiencing severe pain. Pain assessment and reassessment in the elderly requires particular attention due to potential cognitive and physical changes related to age and/or illness severity. These changes may render optimal pain assessment more challenging.
	Utilize the most appropriate pain assessment tool for the individual patient.	Multiple well-validated assessment tools are available. The method of pain assessment should be selected on the basis of the patient's age, developmental stage, and communication and intellectual abilities.	VI: Clinical studies in a variety of populations and situations	See Annotated Bibliography: 1, 5, 6, 7 See Other References: 1, 2, 3, 9, 16, 23, 53 See References: 1, 41, 53	General categories of assessment tools: • Numerical rating scales • Visual analogue scales • Descriptive rating scales
	Establish appropriate frequency of assessment and documentation for selected populations of patients.	The absence or presence of pain should be evaluated and noted in the patient's medical record on a regular basis during acute illness. Unrelieved pain inhibits healing and leads to physiologic complications related to immobility, decrease in pulmonary function, and increased sympathetic response. Unrelieved pain also risks adversarial relationship with caregivers	VI: Clinical studies in a variety of populations and situations	See Other References: 1, 23, 33 See References: 15, 41, 53 See Suggested Readings: 2, 11	See Appendixes 6A and 6B for examples. The most common standard for frequency of assessment of pain in the critical care environment is every 1 to 2 hours. In less acute environments, every 4 to 8 hours is standard. Patients who communicate verbally should be instructed to let a health care provider know when pain is occurring.

Period of Use	Recommendations	Rationale for Recommendation	Level of Recommendation	Supporting References	Comments
Assessment (*cont.*)		and legal liability exposure. Unrelieved pain may also risk development of depression and chronic pain syndromes due to commonality in neurochemical mechanisms.			
	Assess the patient's perception of pain and pain management.	Many patients have misconceptions and fears about pain treatment, especially concerning opioids. Understanding a patient's cultural and sex-related biases about pain is useful in planning pain strategies. Pain tolerance and expressions may also be affected by gender and knowledge base.	IV: Limited clinical studies to support recommendations.	See Other References: 1, 11, 12, 41 See References: 14, 41, 60	Pain expression may be shaped by gender, socialization, and environment. Patient willingness to utilize opioid therapy may be affected by the patient's knowledge base or possible fears of addiction.
Pain Management Interventions	A valid approach to pain management may incorporate the following principles. • Preemptive analgesia is necessary and effective. • Optimal pain management may include interventions that modulate all stages of the pain pathway. This may include interventions at the site of injury such as non-steroidal agents. It may also include modulating the peripheral sensory pathways such as with membrane-stabilizing agents for neuropathic pain. Centrally acting opioid therapy may be utilized to modulate conscious pain perception. Central neuroaxis interventions such as epidural techniques attenuate conduction of pain impulses from the site of injury to higher centers in the brain.	When pain management is planned on the basis of these principles, the entire treatment plan for the patient is enhanced, and optimal outcomes are more likely to be achieved quickly and in a humane manner. Patients state that one of their greatest fears of hospitalization and illness is unrelieved pain. Combining a variety of treatment options is more effective than using only 1 option.	VI: Clinical studies in a variety of populations and situations	See Annotated Bibliography: 2, 3, 4, 8, 10 See Other References: 1, 2, 10, 13, 14, 17, 19, 20, 21, 22, 23, 27, 28, 36, 37, 38, 40, 51, 56, 59, 60, 67 See References: 6, 8, 21, 25, 26, 54, 56, 57 See Suggested Readings: 1, 2, 4, 10, 12	Optimal pain management decreases mortality, morbidity, and length of stay. Patient satisfaction with pain management minimizes opportunities for conflict with health care personnel and decreases legal liability exposure. As such, in addition to providing humane care, patient satisfaction with pain management makes good economic sense for health care providers. There are multiple options for optimal analgesia, all of which incorporate modulation of pain physiology at some level of the pain pathways.

Period of Use	Recommendations	Rationale for Recommendation	Level of Recommendation	Supporting References	Comments
Pain Management Interventions (*cont.*)	Nonpharmacologic methods may be useful adjuncts in pain management and can increase effectiveness of drug therapy, potentially reducing total medication needs.				
	Administer opioid analgesics via the most effective route at the most effective dose for the patient being treated: • IV bolus as needed (appropriate when rapid analgesia or symptom relief is indicated) • IV continuous infusion • Patient controlled analgesia • Transmucosal • Transdermal • Intramuscular • Subcutaneous • Oral or enteral • Epidural • Topical	Many routes of opioid administration are available. Each analgesic regimen should be population, age, and situation appropriate. Physiologic instability of a patient may require opioid dosing with an agent such as fentanyl. It should be administered incrementally and titrated to tolerance and effect. Pain after abdominal, thoracic, or lower extremity procedures may be controlled using epidural techniques. PCA reduces total opioid dosing with improved patient satisfaction. Dosing to effect is of tremendous importance and should be individualized to each patient taking into account pain history and concurrent medications, as many medications may increase tolerance to opioids (including but not limited to opioids and benzodiazepines).	VI: Clinical studies in a variety of patient populations.	See Annotated Bibliography: 4, 10 See Other References: 23, 27, 31, 52 See References: 2, 6, 22, 51, 52 See Suggested Readings: 2, 8	See Appendix 6C for a summary of the selection criteria, advantages, and disadvantages of the most common methods of administration of opioids in the acute and critical care environment.
	Ask health care provider to prescribe specific doses rather than a range of doses.				Clinicians may tend to order or administer the smallest dose when a range of doses is provided. This practice occurs most often with as-needed dosing strategies and often leads to inadequate pain management. Dosage ranges are most appropriately ordered as follows. For mild (pain 1-3/10 scale), moderate (pain 4-6/10 scale), or severe (pain 7-10/10 scale). Reluctance to

Period of Use	Recommendations	Rationale for Recommendation	Level of Recommendation	Supporting References	Comments
Pain Management Interventions (*cont.*)					dose opioids according to patient needs in the presence of tolerance may cause inadequate pain management.
	When changing patients from a parenteral form of opioid administration to an oral form, use equianalgesic dosing charts to assist in selecting the correct dose. These charts are also helpful when changing from one oral opioid to another oral opioid.	The route of administration influences the pharmacokinetics of drugs (absorption, distribution, biotransformation, localization in tissues, elimination). Because of the first-pass effect, patients often have a marked decrease in pain relief if the oral form of a medication is not prescribed in a dose equal (equianalgesic) to the dose they were receiving parenterally.	VI: Clinical studies in a variety of patient populations and situations to support recommendations.	See Other References: 1, 2, 20 See Suggested Readings: 8	Health care providers' misinformation about the relative potency of parenteral and oral preparations contributes to the undertreatment of pain. In general, for oral preparations to achieve potency equal to that of parenteral preparations of the same drug, the oral dose must be much larger than the parenteral dose, because the first-pass effect markedly reduces the circulating level of orally administered preparations. Equianalgesic tables are available in guidelines published by the Agency for Health Care Policy and Research (see Appendix 6C) and the American Pain Society.
	Combine analgesic therapy with treatment of anxiety as clinically appropriate, with slow, incremental titration and close monitoring.	Benzodiazepines are used most often to control anxiety. Pain increases anxiety, and anxiety increases pain perception. When administered concurrently with opioids, benzodiazepines may increase risk of sedation and respiratory depression due to the synergistic effect of combining these drug classes. If used in combination therapy, significantly lower doses should be used initially and titrated slowly to effect.	IV: Limited clinical studies to support recommendations	See Other References: 1, 53 See References: 1, 6, 24, 45 See Suggested Readings: 3, 6, 7, 9	Anxiolytics should be used as an adjunct to, rather than as a substitute for, analgesic medications. Although analgesics may be sedating, they do not have any anxiolytic properties. Conversely, with high-dose benzodiazepine therapy, the patient may be deeply sedated but still experience unrelieved pain and be affected by its hemodynamic and other consequences.
	Combine nonopioid drugs with opioids. Tailor pain management interventions specific to pain physiology.	Nonopioid medications such as acetaminophen and NSAIDs work more effectively in combination therapy. A multimodal approach to pain management utilizing multiple	V: Clinical studies in more than 1 or 2 different populations and situations to support recommendations	See Annotated Bibliography: 3 See Other References: 1, 2, 14, 20, 36, 37, 38, 40, 55, 68 See References: 6, 8, 18, 19, 59	For mild or inflammatory pain, NSAIDs alone or in combination with mild opioids may relieve pain. For severe pain, NSAIDs are effective adjuncts and have an opiate-

Period of Use	Recommendations	Rationale for Recommendation	Level of Recommendation	Supporting References	Comments
Pain Management Interventions (*cont.*)		drug classes may be effective in modulating the central and peripheral pain pathways. Specifically, sodium channel blockers such as lidocaine or other antiarrthymics, anticonvulsants such as phenytoin, carbazepine, neurontin, and tricyclic antidepressant agents all modulate pain physiology and may be particularly effective in managing chronic or neuropathic pain. Also, given the common neurochemical pathways including norepinephrine and serotonin, antidepressants may be effective. Superficial sources of pain such as herpes zoster may respond to topical medications such as lidocaine preparations.			sparing effect. NSAIDs must be used cautiously in the elderly and in patients with a history of hypertension or renal insufficiency. NSAIDs are contraindicated in asthmatics or those at risk for GI bleeding. NSAIDS must be utilized with caution due to potential risk of GI and hematological complications. COX-2 inhibitors specifically may increase risk of cardiovascular and cerebrovascular complications, particularly with long-term use. Using antiarrhythmic and/or anticonvulsant agents to treat neuropathic pain requires close monitoring.
	Use 1 or more of the following nonpharmacologic therapies to increase the effectiveness of the pain management programs: • Instruction of patients on what to expect and on how to assess and decrease pain: • Distraction • Guided imagery • Positioning • Physical supports • Peripheral stimulation (transcutaneous electrical nerve stimulation [TENS] units). Applications of cold or heat, with close monitoring of clinical effects and skin condition may also be utilized. Massage therapy, utilizing techniques including light efflurage and deep tissue massage as appropriate, may be effective.	Most studies on this topic are related to instruction of patients, slow, deep rhythmic/relaxation breathing, relaxation techniques and healing touch.	IV: Limited clinical studies to support recommendations	See Other References: 1, 2, 17, 50, 56, 60	Nonpharmacologic therapies should be used in combination with, rather than instead of, pharmacologic therapies. Most often, the nonpharmacologic therapy can be used after the analgesic medication has been administered and while the patient is waiting for the medication to take effect. See Appendix 6D and Other References 1, 2, and 4 for sample relaxation scripts for use in clinical practice. Additional guidance on this issue may be found in the *Creating a Healing Environment* practice protocol in this series.

Period of Use	Recommendations	Rationale for Recommendation	Level of Recommendation	Supporting References	Comments
Ongoing Monitoring and Evaluation	Pain assessment, interventions, and effectiveness of interventions should be documented at regular intervals to facilitate ongoing evaluation of pain and effectiveness of treatment.	Data on pain and interventions used are needed in order to evaluate the effectiveness of treatments for pain.	V: Clinical studies in more than 1 or 2 different patient populations and situations to support recommendations	See Annotated Bibliography: 5 See Other References: 1, 2, 3, 23, 41, 48, 50, 53, 66 See References: 14, 38, 40 See Suggested Readings: 2, 4, 5, 11	Without consistent documentation, pain at baseline and in response to therapy cannot be evaluated. Many references have sample documentation flowsheets. As clinically appropriate, assessment data should include nonverbal pain behaviors.
	Assess the response to pain medication at the time of onset of action and at the time of peak action: • Oral drugs: 30 minutes and 60 to 90 minutes • Intramuscular drugs: 10 to 15 minutes and 30 to 60 minutes • IV drugs: varies with the drug, usually a few minutes to both onset and peak • Transmucosal drugs: few minutes for onset; peak unknown • Transdermal drugs: varies with the drug; may be several hours to onset and peak	Nurses must assess each patient's response to medication at the time appropriate for the medication and the route of administration. When this practice is followed, medications can be titrated on the basis of peak effect and occurrence of side effects.	VI: Clinical studies in a variety of patient populations and situations to support recommendations.	See Other References: 29 See References: 2, 6, 11, 20, 22 See Suggested Readings: 2, 11	Onset of action is the time when discernible effects of a given medication are expected to begin. Peak action occurs when the maximal effect for a given dose is achieved. At the time of peak action, the side effects of a drug are also at their peak. If a patient is still having marked unrelieved pain at the time of peak action, and no dose-limiting side effects are present, additional doses of the analgesic should be administered. In this way, the nurse titrates the medication to analgesic effects and side effects until pain relief is attained.
Palliative/End-of-Life Care Situations	Pain medications such as opioids should be dosed according to clinical effect for optimal relief of symptoms and suffering.	In end-of-life care situations, aggressive pain/symptom relief is the priority in order to relieve suffering during the dying process. Over time, opioid doses may need to be increased to maintain effective analgesia due to development of tolerance.	IV. Limited clinical studies to support recommendations	See Other References: 21, 35, 42, 49 See References: 10, 28-31, 33, 39, 42, 43	During palliative/end-of-life care situations, priorities have shifted from an aggressive curative approach to an approach focusing on symptom management to relieve suffering. One of the more frequently reported symptoms in ICU survivors is pain and discomfort. Moreover, ICU care is used extensively at the end of life. As such, all personnel involved in caring for patients at end-of-life need to be familiar with all aspects of pain/symptom relief and understand the role of double effect in providing adequate opioid dosing as appropriate

Period of Use	Recommendations	Rationale for Recommendation	Level of Recommendation	Supporting References	Comments
Palliative/End-of-Life Care Situations (*cont.*)					for pain and symptom control. Side effects of opioid therapy such as GI hypomotility, sedation, nausea/vomiting, and possibly delirium/ agitation should be monitored. Bowel programs, close drug titration, and agents to increase GI motility may be options.
Use of Opioid Reversal Agents	For reversal of opioid clinical effects or over-dose, reversal agents should be administered in small incremental doses. Opioid reversal agents may also be utilized to control GI symptoms associated with opioid therapy in acute or critical care settings that have been refractory to other interventions.	Use of opioid reversal agents entails risk of precipitating with-drawal symptoms as well as rebound pain and agitation. There are indications such as with cardiopulmonary compromise when slow titration of opioid reversal agents (nalox-one) may be appropriate to maintain analgesia while preserving cardiorespiratory stability. Opioid side effect of sedation generally precedes that of respiratory depression. Depth of sedation and cardiopulmonary compromise should be used to guide slow, incremental use of opioid reversal agents. In some patients in acute care or ICU settings, GI symptoms such as gastric hypomotility or bowel hypomotility causing constipation or obstruction may occur. Judicious use of reversal agents may be effective in mediating GI symptoms associated with therapy.	IV. Limited clinical studies to support recommendations	See Annotated Bibliography: 9 See References: 6, 11, 17, 22, 51, 56	Acute or emergent administration of naloxone to reverse opioid-associated cardiopulmonary instability can usually be avoided by careful administration of opioids in a controlled incremental manner. If necessary, naloxone (400 μg) should be diluted in 10-20 mL of NSS and administered in 20-40 μg increments to reverse cardiopulmonary compromise associated with opioid use without abruptly reversing analgesia. Using naloxone via the GI tract or IV methylnaltrexone to reverse opioid-induced GI dysfunction or bowel obstruction refractory to other interventions may be an option in a controlled monitored setting.
Managing Side Effects of Prolonged Opioid Administration in Critical Care Settings	For patients requiring opioid infusions, daily interruption of therapy and a protocol-driven approach to drug titration is appropriate to avoid prolonged ventilation times and extended ICU/hospital length of stay.	Prolonged infusions without daily interruption of therapy have been associated with extended ICU length of stay. This risks complications of ICU stay including ventilator-associated pneumonia and airway injury.	V. Clinical studies in more than 1 or 2 different patient populations and situations to support recommendations	See Annotated Bibliography: 2 See Other References: 23 See References: 1, 2, 30, 32, 43, 62 See Suggested Readings: 3, 6, 7, 9	Patents requiring infusions of opioids to control pain or discomfort should be evaluated on an ongoing basis as to the effectiveness of therapy and appropriateness of a daily interruption or downward titration of dose. This facilitates regular

Period of Use	Recommendations	Rationale for Recommendation	Level of Recommendation	Supporting References	Comments
Managing Side Effects of Prolonged Opioid Administration in Critical Care Settings (*cont.*)					neurologic assessment and can result in decreased weaning times, which can facilitate extubation and ICU discharge.

ANNOTATED BIBLIOGRAPHY

1. **Aissauoi Y, Zeggwagh AA, Zekraoui A, et al. Validation of a behavioral pain scale in critically ill, sedated, and mechanically ventilated patients.** *Anesth Analg.* 2005;101(5):1470-1476.

Study Sample
The sample consisted of 360 observations made in 30 critically ill, sedated, and mechanically ventilated patients.

Comparison Studied
Paired observations were evaluated in this study. The psychometric properties studied were reliability, validity, and responsiveness.

Study Procedures
Two observers used the behavioral pain scale (BPS) making 180 observations in 30 patients. The BPS has 3 subscales with a scoring range of 1-4: facial expression, upper limb movements, and compliance with mechanical ventilator.

Key Results
Internal reliability using Cronbach's alpha was .72. Interrater reliability was high (.95), and validity was demonstrated by the significantly higher BPS scores during painful procedures ($P < .001$). The principal components factor analysis indicated a large first factor accounting for 65% of the variance in pain expression. The effect size for responsiveness ranged from 2.2-3.4, indicating excellent responsiveness.

Study Strengths and Weaknesses
The strengths of this study include a factor analysis of validity and the measurement of pain in sedated and ventilated patients experiencing painful procedures. Limitations include inability to generalize results across age groups and patient diagnoses.

Clinical Implications
This tool demonstrates good validity, reliability, and sensitivity to pain assessment in sedated and ventilated patients. It should be compared to other tools to establish superiority.

Without an adequate measure of pain, implementation of pain and sedation algorithms can be difficult.

2. **Dahaba AA, Grabner T, Rehak PH, et al. Remifentanyl versus morphine analgesia and sedation for mechanically ventilated critically ill patients.** *Anesthesiology.* 2004;101(3):640-646.

Study Sample
The study sample consisted of 40 postoperative intent-to-treat patients receiving mechanical ventilation in an intensive care unit.

Comparison Studied
The comparison studied whether and to what degree either morphine infusion or remifentanyl infusion was most effective in terms of outcomes (time to extubation and best quality of sedation/analgesia).

Study Procedures
Forty patients were randomly assigned to receive a blinded infusion of either remifentanyl or morphine. The opioid infusion was titrated to achieve optimal sedation (Sedation-Agitation Scale score of 4). The study was conducted as a controlled, randomized, double-blind, parallel group study. A specific dosing algorithm was followed for all drug dosing (morphine and remifentanyl). Patients were randomly assigned to groups based on a computer-generated randomization list. Randomization was also stratified according to patient acuity. A nurse from the pain clinic prepared the opioid infusions utilized in the study.

Key Results
The mean percentage hours of optimal sedation was significantly longer in the remifentanyl group (78.3 hrs +/- 6.2) than in the morphine group (66.5 hours +/- 8.5) with a P value of .0427. In the remifentanyl group there were less frequent changes in the infusion rate. The mean duration of mechanical ventilation and extubation times were significantly longer in the morphine group (18.1 hours +/- 3.4) versus the remifentanyl group (14.1 hours +/- 2.8) with a P value of .0433. For supplemental sedation, more subjects (n

= 9) required midazolam in the morphine group than in the remifentanyl group (n = 6).

Study Strengths and Weaknesses

Strengths of the study include its design, which minimized bias and controlled for patient acuity. The same dosing algorithm was also used with both the remifentanyl and morphine groups, lending validity to the results.

Weaknesses of the study include sample size and patient type. Results from a sample size of 40 total patients in a postsurgical setting may need to be applied cautiously to a cardiac or medical intensive care population.

Clinical Implications

Clinical implications of this study include that remifentanyl may be a very effective opioid agent for sedation/analgesia in the critically ill population. Chemically related to fentanyl and not requiring end-organ elimination and metabolism, it may contribute to improved outcomes with potentially more widespread use in more ICU populations.

3. Dowling R, Thielmeyer K, Ghaly A, et al. Improved pain control after cardiac surgery: results of a randomized, double-blind clinical trial. *J Thor Cardiovas Surg.* 2003;126(5):1271-1278.

Study Sample

The study sample consisted of 35 cardiac surgical patients at a single medical center. The patients were undergoing either elective coronary artery bypass grafting (CABG) or that combined with laser transmyocardial revascularization.

Comparison Studied

Evaluations of postoperative analgesia effectiveness as measured by narcotic analgesia utilized, mean overall pain scores, mean length of stay, and pulmonary function were compared between an experimental group of patients receiving ropivicaine sternal infusion versus a control group receiving a saline infusion.

Study Procedures

A double-blind, randomized controlled trial was conducted with cardiac surgical patients. At wound closure, 2 catheters with multiple side holes were placed over the sternum. The agent (ropivicaine or saline) was then administered as a regional infusion for 48 hours. Pain assessment scores and systemic narcotic requirements were recorded for 72 hours postoperatively. Secondary outcomes measured included hospital length of stay.

Key Results

The total amount of narcotic required by the ropivicaine group (43.7 mg vs. 78.7 mg) was significantly less (P = .038) than the saline group. The mean overall pain scores

were also less (1.6 vs. 2.6; P = .005) as were length of stay (5.2 vs. 6.3 days; excluding outliers; $P \leq$ .01).

Study Strengths and Weaknesses

Strengths of the study included its design (double-blind and randomized) and the possible confounding lingering effects of anesthesia were controlled for by data collection extending for 72 hours postoperatively. Also, the procedures in question and location/type of intervention were very similar between groups (all required standard median sternotomy) and placement of the infusion catheter was consistent between groups.

Weaknesses of the study included small sample size undergoing a single type of procedure.

Clinical Implications

The data suggest that in cardiac surgical patients, localized infusion of local anesthetics into a surgical bed is effective in improving postoperative analgesia. Given the well-known side effects and risks of high dosing with systemic narcotics, this may be a valid approach with good patient selection. It may facilitate decreased length of stay and lower overall risk associated with prolonged hospitalization.

4. Fulda GJ, Giberson F, Fagracus L. A prospective randomized trial of nebulized morphine compared with patient-controlled analgesia morphine in the management of acute thoracic pain. *J Trauma.* 2005;59(2):382-389.

Study Sample

The sample consisted of 44 patients with posttraumatic thoracic pain randomized into the control group who received nebulized saline every 4 hours and morphine by PCA, and the experimental group who received nebulized morphine every 4 hours and normal saline by PCA.

Comparison Studied

Pulmonary function, pain relief (using a visual analogue scale [VAS]), level of sedation (0-3), total drug administration, and systemic side effects were compared between the 2 groups.

Study Procedures

This double-blind, prospective randomized trial measured the difference between nebulized morphine versus IV morphine delivered through a PCA. Each group had 22 patients, and 770 observations were made. Dose adjustments were made based on the patients' pain responses to the VAS 0-10 pain scale.

Key Results

The 4-hour dose of morphine was significantly higher in the nebulized group (P < .001). However, heart rates were significantly lower in this group (P < .001), and they were less sedated ($P = .02$). There was no difference between pain levels before and after dosing, and the mean pain levels between the groups was not significant. There were no differences between groups in terms of arterial blood pressure, respiratory rate, vital capacity, mean forced expiratory volume in 1 second, spirometric volumes, or SaO_2.

Study Strengths and Weaknesses

The study design is a strength, but the findings are not easily generalized to a population outside of posttraumatic thoracic injury diagnosis. The nebulized morphine was not evaluated in nonverbal patients and during peaks and troughs of pain related to procedures.

Clinical Implications

Nebulized morphine appears to be a safe alternative to standard morphine delivery routes. This route appears to minimize sedation.

5. Odhner M, Wegman D, Freeland N, et al. Assessing pain control in nonverbal critically ill adults. *Dimen Crit Care Nurs.* 2003;22(6):260-267.

Study Sample

A convenience sample of 100 paired (200 individual) assessments obtained by 53 nurses caring for 59 patients over 5 months. Patients admitting diagnoses were trauma, major abdominal surgery, or major burn injury. All patients were unable to speak or self-report level of pain.

Comparison Studied

The study compared individual nurses' paired ratings of pain using 2 nonverbal pain assessment tools: the Face, Legs, Activity, Cry, and Consolability (FLACC) Scale, and the Adult Nonverbal Pain Scale (NVPS).

Study Procedures

Fifty-three nursing staff volunteers agreed to participate. Assessments were made by 2 nurses independently using each of the scales. Assessments were made at periods of rest or when experiencing discomfort during turning or suctioning across all shifts. Each nurse was asked to complete 3 assessments; 26 (49.1%) of the 53 volunteer nurses did.

Key Results

Using Student *t* test, analysis of variance (ANOVA), and chi-square statistical analyses, no difference in rating scores was seen across shifts. Internal consistency reliability measurements (coefficient alpha) were good. A correlation matrix indicated the strongest interscale correlations between the FLACC and NVPS face assessment components (.78); the FLACC legs and NVPS activity components (.72); the FLACC total score and NVPS fact (.71), activity (.71), and guarding components (.69); and the NVPS total

score and the FLACC consolability (.75), legs (.73), activity (.71), and face components (.65). The physiologic II component of the NVPS had the lowest correlation with total score for that scale (.60). The correlation between the total scale scores for the FLACC and NVPS was high (.86).

Study Strengths and Weaknesses

The strength of this study was the comparison of a new nonverbal pain assessment scale with an established gold standard scale. There was good interrater reliability between nurses, and the findings supported the belief that components of the FLACC (designed for use in infants) were not relevant to the adult ICU population.

Limitations included not assessing effects of specific medication peaks and troughs associated with more painful procedural interventions and limited staff involvement.

This study outlines the need for a more refined nonverbal pain assessment tool that can be used in nonverbal critically ill patients. A valid nonverbal pain assessment tool is essential for the safe care and management of critically ill patients. This tool should be compared to the Behavioral Pain Scale used in critically ill sedated and ventilated patients.

6. Pautex S, Herrmann F, LeLous P, et al. Feasibility and reliability of four pain self-assessment scales and correlation with an observational rating scale in hospitalized elderly demented patients. *J Gerontol Biol Sci Med Sci.* 2005; 60(4):524-529.

Study Sample

The sample included 160 acute care and intermediate care patients admitted to a geriatric hospital and consecutively referred to a dementia consultation team.

Comparison Studied

Ratings on 4 unidimensional self-assessment tools were compared to an observational pain rating assessment made independently by the nursing team.

Study Procedures

In this randomized, controlled trial, 4 unidimensional pain tools (verbal, horizontal visual, vertical visual, and faces pain scales) were administered in a randomized fashion to mild, moderate, and severely demented patients. The mean age of patients was 85, and 71% were women. Nurses completed an independent observational pain rating scale.

Key Results

All but 19 (12%) patients could understand at least 1 of the tools (mild dementia, 97%; moderate dementia, 90%; and severe dementia, 40%; $P < .05$). The correlation between the scales is strong (Spearman's $r(s) = 0.81-0.95$; $P < .001$). The observational ratings done by nurses only correlated moderately with the self-assessments and tended to underestimate pain intensity.

Study Strengths and Weaknesses

The study design is a strength. The sample size is relatively small, and there needs to be more correlation with peaks and troughs related to painful procedures.

Clinical Implications

This study indicates that verbal or visual pain scales can be used successfully in demented patients. With the increasing age of the population in acute and critical care, patient self-assessment of pain is possible and should be used over observational pain assessment made by the nurse. Additionally, nonverbal pain assessment is validated, and this has implications for pain assessment applications in the multiple demographics of ICU patient populations where cognitive deficits or other factors interfere with patient interaction.

7. Puntillo KA, Morris AB, Thompson CL, et al. Pain behaviors observed during six common procedures: results from Thunder Project II. *Crit Care Med.* 2004;32(2):421-427.

Study Sample

The sample consisted of a convenience sample comprising 5957 total adult and pediatric patients from multiple units within 169 acute care hospitals in the United States, Canada, England, and Australia.

Comparison Studied

This is an observational study that compared and correlated nonverbal pain behaviors with patients' verbal reports of pain in cognitively intact patients.

Study Procedures

Adult and pediatric patients were included if they were experiencing 1 of the 6 observed procedures (turning, central venous catheter placement, wound drain removal, wound care, tracheal suctioning, and femoral sheath removal). Assessments (verbal and nonverbal indicators) were made at baseline (preprocedure), during the procedure, and postprocedure. Assessments included pain intensity, pain quality, pain location, pain behaviors, and physiologic responses (heart rate and blood pressure). Other information collected included procedural distress, analgesic and sedative profile, use of nonpharmacologic interventions, generic and specific procedure variables, and demographic variables.

Key Results

Pain intensity and distress vary across procedures and age groups. Turning and suctioning were the most distressing procedures for adults. Those with procedural pain were at least 3 times more likely to have behavioral responses than those without procedural pain.

Study Strengths and Weaknesses

Strengths of the study include the large sample size and encompassing a wide variety of diagnoses and a variety of painful procedures experienced by adult and pediatric patients in the study population. Potentially, this makes it easier to generalize the data. Ultimately the most important contribution of the study was in scientifically confirming the relationship between procedural pain and nonverbal cues to acute pain.

Weaknesses of the study include limits on ability to generalize the findings due to the convenience sample and lack of data on specific patients within the population. Effects of long-term sedative or analgesic administration were also limited. There was not standardization of specific interventions for procedural pain. Additionally, with the large number of data collectors and research personnel involved in the study, interrater reliability issues exist with the assessment tool.

Clinical Implications

There is a need to be attentive to repetitive procedures such as turning and suctioning for the potential need for analgesia. Only 6 procedures were studied, and there exist significantly more painful procedures in critical care practice to be evaluated. Future research should be done assessing pain behaviors in a different set of procedures. The findings of this study make it easier to base decisions about potential analgesic administration in cognitively impaired patients using nonverbal pain behaviors (grimacing, increased muscle tension, wincing, clenching fists, etc). Patients should be well prepared for procedures.

8. Story DA, Shelton AC, Poustic SJ, et al. Effect of an anesthesia department led critical care outreach and acute pain service on postoperative serious adverse events. *Anaesthesia.* 2006;61(1):24-28.

Study Sample

The sample in this before-and-after trial consisted of 319 patients before the project implementation and 271 patients following the project implementation. All were high-risk surgical patients who returned to the general ward.

Comparison Studied

The effect of an anesthesia-led critical care pain outreach program on postoperative adverse events was evaluated in patients returning to the general ward.

Study Procedures

A critical care outreach and acute pain service programs were combined into an inpatient management of acute pain and advice on clinical treatment program (IMPACT) led by the anesthesia department. The incidence of adverse postoperative events was compared preimplementation of the program to postimplementation. Patients were followed by the team for 3 days after surgery.

Key Results

The incidence of serious adverse events decreased from 23 events per 100 patients to 16 events per 100 patients. The 30-day mortality decreased from 9% to 3% (P = .004).

Study Strengths and Weaknesses

A prospective pre- and post-trial of evaluating a new monitoring program is a strength. The limitations are that the study is done in a different type of health system than found in the United States, and the patient population is all acute versus critical care.

Clinical Implications

In this era of cost containment and patient safety, more creative programs such as this need to be evaluated. The results seem impressive. Good screening and adequate resources for specialty-specific follow-up monitoring may prove to effectively decrease use of intermediate and critical care beds while maintaining patient safety in a select group of patients.

9. **Yuan CS, Foss JF, O'Connor M, et al. Methylnaltrexone for reversal of constipation due to chronic methadone use: a randomized controlled trial.** *JAMA.* **2000;283(3):367-372.**

Study Sample

The study sample consisted of 22 subjects (9 men and 13 women) enrolled in a methadone maintenance program and having methadone-induced constipation.

Comparison Studied

Comparisons of laxation response, oral-cecal transit time, and central opioid withdrawal symptoms were compared between the placebo versus the methylnaltrexone group.

Study Procedures

This is a double-blind, randomized, placebo-controlled trial. Subjects were randomly assigned to either the placebo or the methylnaltrexone groups. Neither the patients nor those administering the medications (placebo versus methylnaltrexone) were aware of which was being administered. Laxation response, oral-cecal transit time, and presence/degree of central opioid withdrawal symptoms were compared between the 2 groups.

Key Results

The 11 patients in the placebo group showed no laxation response, and all 11 patients in the methylnaltrexone group showed laxation response following IV methylnaltrexone administration. Specifically, the oral-cecal transit times deceased significantly (by 77.7 minutes; *P* ≤ .001) in the methylnaltrexone group as compared to a decrease of 1.4

minutes; (*P* ≤ .001) in the placebo group. None of the subjects experienced systemic opioid withdrawal, and no significant adverse effects were reported by any of the study subjects.

Study Strengths and Weaknesses

Strengths of the study included its design of a double-blind, randomized, placebo-controlled study significantly controlling for any possible bias in the results as well as eliminating altered results due to a placebo effect.

Weaknesses of the study include the small sample size (22 patients) from which it may be problematic to draw sweeping conclusions. Moreover, the subjects studied were experiencing GI hypomotility only related to chronic methadone use and not other systemic opioid therapies such as morphine or transdermal fentanyl. Attempts to generalize results from this study to other populations should be done cautiously for these reasons.

Clinical Implications

GI hypomotility as a side effect of opioid therapy has implications for patient outcomes and may lead to aspiration, ileus, constipation/bowel obstruction, as well as compromised ability to provide optimal nutritional support. Validation of interventions to more effectively control GI complications of systemic opioid therapy may offer alternatives to improve GI function in patients utilizing systemic opioid therapy.

10. **Zeppetella G. An assessment of the safety, efficacy and acceptability of intranasal fentanyl citrate in the management of cancer-related breakthrough pain: a pilot study.** *J Pain Symp Mgmt.* **2000;20(4):253-258.**

Study Sample

The study sample consisted of 12 hospice inpatients with cancer-related breakthrough pain.

Comparison Studied

The patients served as their own controls, having long pain histories related to their cancer diagnosis. Their previous pain histories, including incidence of breakthrough pain, and the effectiveness of prior interventions such as oral morphine preparations were documented. They were enrolled, and the effectiveness of intranasal transmucosal fentanyl citrate for managing breakthrough pain was compared with prior interventions.

Study Procedures

Following enrollment and informed consent, a record was made of both chronic and breakthrough pain experienced by the patient, analgesic use, and analgesic effectiveness. Patients were chosen who were experiencing nociceptive rather than neuropathic pain. During episodes of breakthrough pain, fentanyl citrate was administered via spray bottles delivering 0.2 mL/20 µg fentanyl citrate per adminis-tration. Pain was assessed with the visual analog scale and measured at 3, 5, 10, 15, 30, 45, and 60 minutes following intervention. Maintenance analgesics were continued.

Key Results

Most patients reported the intervention was effective, and 9 out of 12 patients would have continued the treatment if it were available.

Study Strengths and Weaknesses

Strengths of the study included using the patient as their own control. The patients in the study were cognitively intact and very familiar with their illness and all related ther-apies. Also, effectiveness of the intervention was assessed by the patient's verbal report, which is considered the gold standard for pain assessment.

Weaknesses of the study included that 9 out of 12 patients were men, skewing the frequency distribution of gender. Sex-related differences do exist in pain responses, and this may not have been reflected by the gender mix of the study sample. Sample size is small but identified as a pilot study.

Clinical Implications

Most drug (analgesic) administration in critically ill patients is by IV bolus or infusion dosing. There are circumstances such as end-of-life and palliative care situations or other sit-uations where, if IV access is not available, validation of a less painful and less invasive route of administration can improve practice by identifying appropriate alternatives to IV administration.

OTHER REFERENCES

1. Agency for Health Care Policy and Research. *Acute Pain Management: Operative or Medical Procedures and Trauma* [clinical practice guideline 1]. Rockville, Md: US Dept of Health and Human Services; 1992. Agency for Health Care Policy and Research publica-tion 92-0032.

2. Agency for Health Care Policy and Research. *Manage-ment of Cancer Pain* [clinical practice guideline 9]. Rockville, Md: US Dept of Health and Human Services; 1994. Agency for Health Care Policy and Research pub-lication 94-0592.

3. Aissauoi Y, Zeggwagh AA, Zekraoui A, et al. Valida-tion of a behavioral pain scale in critically ill, sedated, and mechanically ventilated patients. *Anesth Analg.* 2005;101(5):1470-1476.

4. Angus DE, Barnato AE, Linde-Zeirble WT, et al. Use of intensive care at the end of life in the United States: an epidemiologic study. *Crit Care Med.* 2004;32(3): 638-643.

5. Arbour R. Mastering neuromuscular blockade. *Dimens Crit Care Nurs.* 2000;19(5):4-18.

6. Arbour R. Using the bispectral index to assess arousal response in a patient with neuromuscular blockade. *Am J Crit Care.* 2000;9(6):383-387.

7. Arbour R. Monitoring the nervous system: EEG, the bispectral index and neuromuscular transmission. *AACN Clin Iss.* 2003;14(2):185-207.

8. Burgess FW. Innovations in practice: cell therapy for can-cer pain management. *Am Pain Soc Bull.* Available at: http://www.ampainsoc.org/pub/bulletin/nov96/innovations. htm. Accessed October 16, 2001.

9. Carroll KC, Atkin PJ, Herold GR, et al. Pain assessment and management in critically ill postoperative and trauma patients: a multisite study. *Am J Crit Care.* 1999;8(2):105-117.

10. Carson M, Barton D, Morrison C, et al. Managing pain during mediastinal chest tube removal. *Heart Lung.* 1994;23:500-505.

11. Chen W, Woods SL, Wilkie DJ, Puntillo KA. Gender differences in symptom experiences of patients with acute coronary syndromes. *J Pain Symptom Manage.* 2005;30(6):553-562.

12. Chen W, Woods SL, Puntillo KA. Gender differences in symptoms associated with acute myocardial infarction: a review of the research. *Heart Lung.* 2005;34(4):240-247.

13. Cleary JF. Cancer pain management. *Cancer Control.* 2000;7(2):120-131.

14. Dworkin RH, Backojna M, Rowbotham MC, et al. Advances in neuropathic pain: diagnosis, mechanisms and treatment recommendations. *Arch Neurol.* 2003; 60(11):1524-1534.

15. Graf C, Puntillo K. Pain in the older adult in the inten-sive care unit. *Crit Care Clin.* 2003;19(4):749-770.

16. Gujol M. A survey of pain assessment and management practices among critical care nurses. *Am J Crit Care.* 1994;3:123-128.

17. Hader CF, Guy J. Your hand in pain management. *Nurs Manag.* 2004;35(11):21-27.

18. Hagen NA, Elwood T, Ernst S. Cancer pain emergen-cies: a protocol for management. *J Pain Symp Manag.* 1997;14(1):45-50.

19. Hall JE, Uhrich TD, Ebert TJ. Sedative, analgesic and cognitive effects of clonidine infusions in humans. *Br J Anaest.* 2001;86(1):5-11.

20. Hauer M, Cram E, Titler M, et al. Intravenous patient-controlled analgesia in critically ill postoperative/ trauma patients: research-based practice recommenda-tions. *Dimens Crit Care Nurs.* 1995;14:144-153.

21. Herndon CM. Pharmacologic management of cancer pain. *J Neurosci Nurs.* 2003;35(6):321-326.

22. Horgas AL, McLennon SM. Pain management. In: Mezey M, Fulmer T, Abraham I, Zwicker DA, eds. *Geri-atric Nursing Protocols for Best Practice.* 2nd ed. New York, NY: Springer Publishing Co Inc; 2003:229-250.

23. Jacobi J, Fraser GL, Coursin DB, et al. Clinical practice

guidelines for the sustained use of sedatives and analgesics in the critically ill adult. *Crit Care Med.* 2002; 30(1):119-141.

24. Kumar K, Hunter G, Demeria DD. Treatment of chronic pain by using intrathecal drug delivery compared with conventional pain therapies: A cost-effectiveness analysis. *J Neurosurg.* 2002:97(4);803-810.

25. Lawrence M. The unconscious experience. *Am J Crit Care.* 1995;4:227-232.

26. Lindaman C. Talking to physicians about pain control. *Am J Nurs.* 1995;95(1):36-37.

27. Liu LL, Gropper MA. Postoperative analgesia and sedation in the adult intensive care unit: a guide to drug selection. *Drugs.* 2003;63(8):755-767.

28. Luketich JD, Land SR, Sullivan EA, et al. Thoracic epidural versus intercostal nerve catheter plus patient-controlled analgesia: a randomized study. *Ann Thorac Surg.* 2005;79(6):1845-1849; discussion 1849-1850.

29. McKenry L, Salerno E. *Mosby's Pharmacology in Nursing.* 22nd ed. St Louis, Mo: CV Mosby; 2005.

30. Mancini I, Dumon JC, Body JJ. Efficacy and safety of ibandronate in the treatment of opioid-resistant bone pain associated with metastatic bone disease: a pilot study. *J Clin Oncol.* 2004;22:3587-3592.

31. Marlowe KF, Chicella MF. Treatment of sickle cell pain. *Pharmacotherapy.* 2002;22(4):484-491.

32. Maxam-Moore V, Wilkie D, Woods S. Analgesics for cardiac surgery patients in critical care: describing current practice. *Am J Crit Care.* 1994;3:31-39.

33. Miaskowski C. Recent advances in understanding pain mechanisms provide future directions for pain management. *Oncol Nurs Forum.* 2004;31(4 suppl):25-35.

34. Myles P, Buckland M, Cannon G, et al. Comparison of patient-controlled analgesia and nurse-controlled infusion analgesia after cardiac surgery. *Anaesth Intensive Care.* 1994;22:672-678.

35. Nelson JE, Meier DE, Oei EJ, et al. Self-reported symptom experience of critically ill cancer patients receiving intensive care. *Crit Care Med.* 2001;29(2):277-282.

36. Pandey CK, Singhal V, Kumar M, et al. Gabapentin provides effective postoperative analgesia whether administered pre-emptively or not. *Can J Anaesth.* 2005; 52(8):827-831.

37. Pandey CK, Raza M, Tripathi M, et al. The comparative evaluation of gabapentin and carbamazepime for pain management in Guillain-Barre syndrome patients in the intensive care unit. *Anesth Analg.* 2005;101(1):220-225.

38. Pandey CK, Navkar DV, Giri PJ, et al. Evaluation of the optimal preemptive dose of gabapentin for postoperative pain relief after lumbar diskectomy: a randomized, double-blind, placebo-controlled study. *J Neurosurg Anesthes.* 2005;17(2):65-68.

39. Pandey CK, Raza M, Ranjan R, et al. Intravenous lidocaine 0.5 mg.kg-1 effectively suppresses fentanyl-induced cough. *Can J Anaesth.* 2005;52(2):172-175.

40. Pettersson PH, Jakobsson J, Owall A. Intravenous acetaminophen reduced the use of opioids compared with oral administration after coronary artery bypass grafting. *J Cardiothorac Vasc Anesth.* 2005;19(3): 306-309.

41. Pettersson PH, Settergren G, Owall A. Similar pain scores after early and late extubation in heart surgery with cardiopulmonary bypass. *J Cardiothorac Vasc Anesth.* 2004;18(1):64-67.

42. Prendergast TJ, Puntillo KA. Withdrawal of life support: intensive caring at the end of life. *JAMA.* 2002; 288(21):2732-2740.

43. Puntillo K, Weiss S. Pain: its mediators and associated morbidity in critically ill cardiovascular surgical patients. *Nurs Res.* 1994;43:31-36.

44. Puntillo K. Dimensions of procedural pain and its analgesic management in critically ill surgical patients. *Am J Crit Care.* 1994;3:116-122.

45. Puntillo KA, White C, Morris AB, et al. Patients' perceptions and responses to procedural pain: results from Thunder Project II. *Am J Crit Care.* 2001;10(4):238-251.

46. Puntillo KA, Wild LR, Morris AB, et al. Practices and predictors of analgesic interventions for adults undergoing painful procedures. *Am J Crit Care.* 2002;11(5):415-429.

47. Puntillo KA, Stannard D, Miaskowski C, et al. Use of a pain assessment and intervention notation (P. A. I. N.) tool in critical care nursing practice: nurses' observations. *Heart Lung.* 2002;31(4):303-314.

48. Rakel B, Herr K. Assessment and treatment of postoperative pain in older adults. *J Perianesth Nurs.* 2004; 19(3):194-208.

49. Rotondi AJ, Chelluri L, Sirio C, et al. Patients' recollections of stressful experiences while receiving prolonged mechanical ventilation in an intensive care unit. *Crit Care Med.* 2002;30(4):746-752.

50. Schmidt K, Alpen M, Rakel B. Implementation of the Agency for Health Care Policy and Research pain guidelines. *AACN Clin Issues Adv Pract Acute Care.* 1996;7:425-435.

51. Schultz-Stubner S, Boezaart A, Hata JS. Regional analgesia in the critically ill. *Crit Care Med.* 2005;33(6): 1400-1407.

52. Searle N, Roy M, Gergeron G, et al. Hydromorphone patient-controlled analgesia after coronary bypass surgery. *Can J Anaesth.* 1994;41:198-205.

53. Stanik-Hutt J. Acute pain: clinical application of pain management. In: Salerno E, Willens J, eds. *Pain Management Handbook: An Interdisciplinary Approach.* St Louis, Mo: Mosby; 1996:233-272.

54. Stanik-Hutt JA, Soeken KL, Belcher AE, et al. Pain experiences of traumatically injured patients in a critical care setting. *Am J Crit Care.* 2001;10(4):252-259.

55. Stanik-Hutt JA. Management options for angina refractory to maximal medical and surgical interventions. *AACN Clin Issues.* 2005;16(3):320-332.

56. Stephenson NL, Dalton JA. Using reflexology for pain management: a review. *J Holist Nurs.* 2003;21(2): 179-191.

57. Stotts NA, Puntillo K, Bonham-Morris A, et al. Wound care pain in hospitalized adult patients. *Heart Lung.* 2004;33(5):321-332.

58. Sullivan FL, Muir MR, Ginsberg B. A survey on the clinical use of epidural catheters for acute pain management. *J Pain Symptom Manage.* 1994;9:303-307.

59. Summer GJ, Puntillo KA. Management of surgical and procedural pain in a critical care setting. *Crit Care Nurs Clin North Am.* 2001;13(2):233-242.

60. Thomas EM, Weiss SM. Nonpharmacological interventions with chronic cancer pain in adults. *Cancer Control.* 2000;7(2):157-164.

61. Thompson CL, White C, Wild LR, et al. Translating research into practice: implications of the Thunder Project II. *Crit Care Nurs Clin North Am.* 2001;13(4): 541-546.

62. Titler MG, Herr K, Schilling ML, et al. Acute pain treatment for older adults hospitalized with hip fracture: current nursing practices and perceived barriers. *Appl Nurs Res.* 2003;16(4):211-227.

63. Tittle M, MacMillan SC. Pain and pain-related side effects in an ICU and on a surgical unit: nurses' management. *Am J Crit Care.* 1994;3:25-30.

64. Ulmer J. Identifying and preventing pain mismanagement. In: Salerno E, Willens J, eds. *Pain Management Handbook: An Interdisciplinary Approach.* St Louis, Mo: Mosby; 1996:39-66.

65. Valdix S, Puntillo K. Pain, pain relief and accuracy of their recall after cardiac surgery. *Prog Cardiovasc Nurs.* 1995;10(3):3-11.

66. Young G, Siffleet J, Nikoletti S, Shaw T. Use of a behavioural pain scale to assess pain in ventilated, unconscious and/or sedated patients. *Intensive Crit Care Nurs.* 2006;22(1):32-39.

67. Dowling R, Thielmeier K, Ghaly A, Barber D, Boice T, Dine A. Improved pain control after cardiac surgery: results of a randomized, double-blind, clinical trial. *J Thor Cardiovasc Surg.* 2003;126(5):1271-1278.

68. Guay DRP. Adjunctive agents in the management of chronic pain. *Pharmacotherapy.* 2001; 21(99):1071-1081.

69. Soifer BE. Procedural anesthesia at the bedside. *Crit Care Clin.* 2000;16(1):7-28.

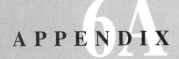

Pain Assessment Scales

Figure 6A-1: Simple pain assessment scales for adults

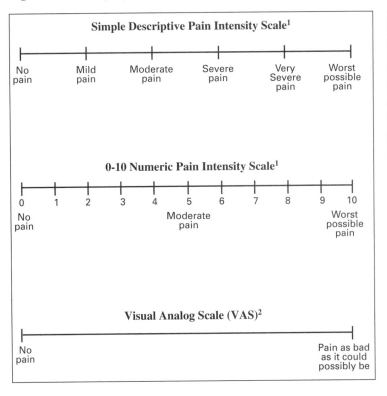

Figure 6A-2: Pain intensity scales

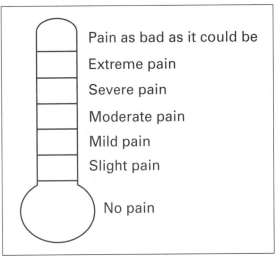

Reprinted with permission from Herr K, Mobily P. Comparison of selected pain assessment tools for use with the elderly. *Appl Nurs Res.* 1993;6:39-46.

[1]If used as a graphic rating scale, a 10-cm baseline is recommended.

[2]A 10-cm baseline is recommended for VAS scales.

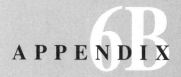
Adult Nonverbal Pain Scale

Categories	0	1	2
Face	No particular expression or smile	Occasional grimace, tearing, frowning, wrinkled forehead	Frequent grimace, tearing, frowning, wrinkled forehead
Activity (Movement)	Lying quietly, normal position	Seeking attention through movement or slow, cautious movement	Restless, excessive activity, and/or withdrawal reflexes
Guarding	Lying quietly, no positioning of hands over areas of body	Splinting areas of the body, tense	Rigid, stiff
Physiology (vital signs)	Stable vital signs	Change in any of the following: SBP > 20 mmHg, HR > 20/minute	Change in any of the following: SBP > 30 mm Hg, HR> 25/minute
Respiratory	Baseline RR/S_pO_2 compliant with ventilator	RR > 10 above baseline, or 5% ↓ S_pO_2 mild asynchrony with ventilator	RR > 20 above baseline or 10% ↓ S_pO_2 severe asynchrony with ventilator

Abbreviations: HR, heart rate; RR, respiratory rate; SBP, systolic blood pressure; S_pO_2, pulse oximetry

Instructions: Each of the 5 categories is scored from 0-2, which results in a total score between 0 and 10. Document total score by adding numbers from each of the 5 categories. Scores of 0-2 indicate no pain, 3-6 moderate pain, and 7-10 severe pain. Document assessment every 4 hours on nursing flowsheet and complete assessment before and after intervention to maximize patient comfort. Sepsis, hypovolemia, hypoxia need to be excluded before interventions.

Source: Strong Memorial Hospital, University of Rochester Medical Center, 2004. Used with permission

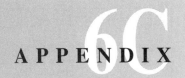

Commonly Used Opioid and NSAID Analgesics and Dosing Data for Opioid Analgesics*

Table 6C-1   Dosing Data for Opioid Analgesics in Adults

Drug	Approximate equianalgesic oral dose	Approximate equianalgesic parenteral dose	Recommended starting dose (adults more than 50 kg body weight)		Recommended starting dose (children and adults less than 50 kg body weight)	
			Oral	Parenteral	Oral	Parenteral
Opioid Agonist						
Morphine[2]	30 mg every 3-4 hr (around-the-clock dosing); 60 mg every 3-4 hr (single dose or intermittent dosing)	10 mg every 3-4 hr	30 mg every 3-4 hr	10 mg every 3-4 hr	0.3 mg/kg every 3-4 hr	0.1 mg/kg every 3-4 hr
Codeine[2]	130 mg every 3-4 hr	75 mg every 3-4 hr	60 mg every 3-4 hr	60 mg every 2 hr (intramuscular/subcutaneous)	1 mg/kg every 3-4 hr[4]	Not recommended
Hydromophone[2] (Dilaudid)	7.5 mg every 3-4 hr	1.5 mg every 3-4 hr	6 mg every 3-4 hr	1.5 mg every 3-4 hr	0.06 mg/kg every 3-4 hr	0.015 mg/kg every 3-4 hr
Hydrocodone (in Lorcet, Lortab, Vicodin, others)	30 mg every 3-4 hr	Not available	10 mg every 3-4 hr	Not available	0.2 mg/kg every 3-4 hr[4]	Not available
Levorphanol (Levo-Dromoran)	4 mg every 6-8 hr	2 mg every 6-8 hr	4 mg every 6-8 hr	2 mg every 6-8 hr	0.04 mg/kg every 6-8 hr	0.02 mg/kg every 6-8 hr
Meperidine (Demerol)	300 mg every 2-3 hr	100 mg every 2-3 hr	Not recommended	100 mg every 3 hr	Not recommended	0.75 mg/kg every 2-3 hr
Methadone (Dolophine, others)	20 mg every 6-8 hr	10 mg every 6-8 hr	20 mg every 6-8 hr	10 mg every 6-8 hr	0.2 mg/kg every 6-8 hr	0.1 mg/kg every 6-8 hr
Oxycodone (Roxicodone, also in Percocet, Percodan, Tylox, others)	30 mg every 3-4 hr	Not available	10 mg every 3-4 hr	Not available	0.2 mg/kg every 3-4 hr[4]	Not available
Oxymorphone[2] (Numorphan)	Not available	1 mg every 3-4 hr	Not available	1 mg every 3-4 hr	Not recommended	Not recommended

*Other References: 1.

(continued)

Table 6C-1   Dosing Data for Opioid Analgesics in Adults (*cont.*)

Drug	Approximate equianalgesic oral dose	Approximate equianalgesic parenteral dose	Recommended starting dose (adults more than 50 kg body weight)		Recommended starting dose (children and adults less than 50 kg body weight)	
			Oral	Parenteral	Oral	Parenteral
Opioid Agonist-Antagonist and Partial Agonist						
Buprenorphine (Buprenex)	Not available	0.3-0.4 mg every 6-8 hr	Not available	0.4 mg every 6-8 hr	Not available	0.004 mg/kg every 6-8 hr
Butorphanol (Stadol)	Not available	2 mg every 3-4 hr	Not available	2 mg every 3-4 hr	Not available	Not recommended
Nalbuphine (Nubain)	Not available	10 mg every 3-4 hr	Not available	10 mg every 3-4 hr	Not available	0.1 mg/kg every 3-4 hr
Pentazocine (Talwin, others)	150 mg every 3-4 hr	60 mg every 3-4 hr	50 mg every 4-6 hr	Not recommended	Not recommended	Not recommended

Note: Published tables vary in the suggested doses that are equianalgesic to morphine. Clinical response is the criterion that must be applied for each patient; titration to clinical response is necessary. Because there is not complete cross tolerance among these drugs, it is usually necessary to use a lower than equianalgesic dose when changing drugs and to retitrate response.

Caution: Recommended doses do not apply to patients with renal or hepatic insufficiency or other conditions affecting drug metabolism and kinetics.

1. **Caution:** Doses listed for patients with body weight less than 50 kg cannot be used as initial starting doses in babies less than 6 months of age. Consult the *Clinical Practice Guideline for Acute Pain Management: Operative or Medical Procedures and Trauma* section on management of pain in neonates for recommendations.

2. For morphine, hydromorphone, and oxymorphone, rectal administration is an alternate route for patients unable to take oral medications, but equianalgesic doses may differ from oral and parenteral doses because of pharmacokinetic differences.

3. **Caution:** Codiene doses above 65 mg are often not appropriate due to diminishing incremental analgesia with increasing doses but continually increasing constipation and other side effects.

4. **Caution:** Doses of aspirin and acetaminophen in combination with opiod/NSAID preparations must also be adjusted to the patient's body weight.

Table 6C-2   Dosing Data for Opioid Analgesics in Children

Drug	Usual adult dose	Usual pediatric dose[1]	Comments
Oral NSAIDs			
Acetaminophen	650-975 mg every 4 hr	10-15 mg/kg every 4 hr	Acetaminophen lacks the peripheral anti-inflammatory activity of other NSAIDs
Aspirin	650-975 mg every 4 hr[2]	10-15 mg/kg every 4 hr	The standard against which other NSAIDS are compared. Inhibits platelet aggregation; may cause postoperative bleeding
Choline magnesium trisalicylate (Trilsate)	1000-1500 mg bid	25 mg/kg bid	May have minimal antiplatelet activity; also available as oral liquid
Diflunisal (Dolobid)	1000 mg initial dose followed by 500 mg every 12 hr		
Etodolac (Lodine)	200-400 mg every 6-8 hr		
Fenoprophen calcium (Nalfon)	200 mg every 4-6 hr		
Ibuprophen (Motrin)	400 mg every 4-6 hr	10 mg/kg every 6-8 hr	Available as several brand names and as generic; also available as oral suspension
Ketoprophen (Orudis)	25-75 mg every 6-8 hr		
Magnesium salicylate	650 mg every 4 hr		Many brands and generic forms available
Meclofenamate sodium (Meclomen)	50 mg every 4-6 hr		
Mefenamic acid (Ponstel)	250 mg every 6 hr		

Note: Only the above NSAIDs have FDA approval for use as simple analgesics, but clinical experience has been gained with other drugs as well.

1. Drug recommendations are limited to NSAIDs where pediatric dosing experience is available.

2. Contraindicated in presence of fever or other evidence of viral illness.

Table 6C-2   Dosing Data for Opioid Analgesics in Children (*cont.*)

Drug	Usual adult dose	Usual pediatric dose[1]	Comments
Oral NSAIDs (*cont.*)			
Naproxen (Naprosyn)	500 mg initial dose followed by 250 mg every 6-8 hr	5 mg/kg every 12 hr	Also available as an oral liquid
Naproxen sodium (Anaprox)	550 mg initial dose followed by 275 mg every 6-8 hr		
Salsalate (Disalcid, others)	500 mg every 4 hr		May have minimal antiplatelet activity
Sodium salicylate	325-650 mg every 3-4 hr		Available in generic form from several distributors
Parenteral NSAID			
Ketorolac tromethamine (Toradol)	30 or 60 mg IM initial dose followed by 15 or 30 mg every 6 hr. Oral dose following IM dosage: 10 mg every 6-8 hr		Intramuscular dosage not to exceed 5 days

Note: Only the above NSAIDs have FDA approval for use as simple analgesics, but clinical experience has been gained with other drugs as well.

1. Drug recommendations are limited to NSAIDs where pediatric dosing experience is available.

From Agency for Health Care Policy and Research. *Acute Pain Management: Operative or Medical Procedures and Trauma* [clinical practice guideline 1]. Rockville, Md: US Dept of Health and Human Services; 1992. Agency for Health Care Policy and Research publication 92-0032.

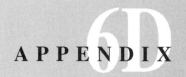

Relaxation Scripts

EXERCISE 1: SLOW RHYTHMIC BREATHING FOR RELAXATION

1. Breathe in slowly and deeply.
2. As you breathe out slowly, feel yourself beginning to relax; feel the tension leaving your body.
3. Now breathe in and out slowly and regularly, at whatever rate is comfortable for you. You may wish to try abdominal breathing.
4. To help you focus on your breathing and breathe slowly and rhythmically: (a) breathe in as you say silently to yourself, "in, two, three"; (b) breathe out as you say silently to yourself, "out, two, three."

   Or, each time you breathe out, say silently to yourself a word such as "peace" or "relax."
5. Do steps 1 through 4 only once, or repeat steps 3 and 4 for up to 20 minutes.
6. End with a slow deep breath. As you breathe out say to yourself, "I feel alert and relaxed."

EXERCISE 2: SIMPLE TOUCH, MASSAGE, OR WARMTH FOR RELAXATION

Touch and massage are age-old methods of helping others relax. Some examples are

- Brief touch or massage, such as handholding or briefly touching or rubbing a person's shoulder
- Offer a warm foot soak in a basin of warm water, or wrap the feet in a warm, wet towel.
- Massage (3 to 10 minutes) may consist of the whole body or be restricted to back, feet, or hands. If the patient is modest or cannot move or turn easily in bed, consider massage of the hands and feet.
  - Use a warm lubricant. For example, a small bowl of hand lotion may be warmed in the microwave oven, or a bottle of lotion may be warmed by placing it in a sink of hot water for about 10 minutes.
- Massage for relaxation is usually done with smooth, long, slow strokes. (Rapid strokes, circular movements, and squeezing of tissues tend to stimulate circulation and increase arousal.) However, try several degrees of pressure along with different types of massage, for example, kneading, stroking, and circling. Determine which is preferred.

Especially for the elderly, a back rub that effectively produces relaxation may consist of no more than 3 minutes of slow, rhythmic stroking (about 60 strokes per minute) on both sides of the spinous process from the crown of the head to the lower back. Continuous hand contact is maintained by starting one hand down the back as the other hand stops at the lower back and is raised. Set aside a regular time for the massage. This practice gives the patient something to look forward to and depend on.

EXERCISE 3: PEACEFUL PAST EXPERIENCES

Something may have happened to you a while ago that brought you peace and comfort. You may be able to draw on the past experience to bring you peace and comfort now. Think about these questions:

1. Can you remember any situation, even when you were a child, when you felt calm, peaceful, secure, hopeful, or comfortable?
2. Have you ever daydreamed about something peaceful? What were you thinking of?
3. Do you get a dreamy feeling when you listen to music? Do you have any favorite music?

4. Do you have any favorite poetry that you find uplifting or reassuring?

5. Have you ever been religiously active? Do you have favorite readings, hymns, or prayers? Even if you haven't heard or thought of them for many years, childhood religious experiences may still be very soothing.

Additional points: Very likely some of the things you think of in answer to these questions can be recorded for you, such as your favorite music or a prayer. Then, you can listen to the tape whenever you wish. Or, if your memory is strong, you may simply close your eyes and recall the events or words.

EXERCISE 4: ACTIVE LISTENING TO RECORDED MUSIC

1. Obtain the following:
- A cassette player or tape recorder; small, battery-operated ones are more convenient.
- Earphone or headset; this is a more demanding stimulus than a speaker a few feet away, and it avoids disturbing others.
- Cassette of music you like; most people prefer fast, lively music, but some select relaxing music. Other options are comedy routines, sporting events, old radio show, or stories.

2. Mark time to the music. For example, tap out the rhythm with your finger or nod your head. This practice helps you concentrate on the music rather than on your discomfort.

3. Keep your eyes open and focus steadily on one stationary spot or object. If you wish to close your eyes, picture something about the music.

4. Listen to the music at a comfortable volume. If the discomfort increases, try increasing the volume; decrease the volume when the discomfort decreases.

5. If this is not effective enough, try adding or changing one or more of the following: massage your body in rhythm to the music; try other music; mark time to the music in more than one manner, for example, tap your foot and finger at the same time.

Additional points: Many patients have found this technique helpful. It tends to be popular, probably because the equipment is usually readily available and is part of daily life. Other advantages are that it is easy to learn and is not physically or mentally demanding. If you are very tired, you may simply listen to the music and omit marking time or focusing on a spot.

Source: McCaffery M, Beedbe A. *Pain: Clinical Manual for Nursing Practice.* St Louis, Mo: CV Mosby; 1989:177,201,206,207.